Praise for *The Gentle Sleep Book*

'Sleep is so crucial to our wellbeing, and so precious when our children are young. This is why it has become such a contentious issue among parenting writers and experts. In *The Gentle Sleep Book*, Sarah Ockwell-Smith starts by looking at scientific, cultural and historical perspectives and so allows us to put sleep in context. Her central message is that children don't have sleep problems, we as a society have created expectations and demands of parenting that are not in harmony with a child's biological or psychological needs and then struggle when children don't sleep as we "need" them to.

I like the perspective Sarah takes, the position of trying to make parents feel informed and supported rather than criticised. Sleep is not a battle, it's a balance and in this reassuring book Sarah helps parents find that balance. At the end of the book are emails from parents with advice Sarah has shared using her BEDTIME acronym – Bedsharing and co-sleeping; Expectations; Diet; Transitional objects: IT and Screen time; Me-time and Environment. I think this section of practical advice for real situations is very helpful. In these modern times new parents are isolated and struggling to manage alone. Often Sarah's advice is not to fight your child's sleep pattern but to try and find help for yourself so that you are better able to cope. This, I think, is a wonderful gentle message that would benefit many aspects of family life.'

Saffia Farr, Editor, *JUNO* magazine

'This book is a wonderful blend of science and wisdom. Using the latest scientific research as a foundation, Sarah teaches families how to use a responsive and nurturing hand to guide babies and toddlers into age-appropriate sleep. It will help parents develop realistic expectations about the course of their infant's sleep development, giving them reassurance and the confidence to use the specific strategies provided in a way that it is just right for their child.'

Sara Pearce RN CNM IBCLC
CEO, Director of Education,
Amma Parenting Center

'This book should be called The Sleep *Bible* and needs to be in every parent's bedside drawer. As always, Sarah Ockwell-Smith has written a book that is easy to read and jam-packed with refreshing new ideas to help little ones relax and sleep, and to help parents reduce their dark circles and eye bags!'

Marneta Viegas, founder of Relax Kids – classes, books
and CDs to help children relax, manage
anxiety and stress, and sleep

THE
GENTLE
SLEEP BOOK

A guide for

CALM BABIES, TODDLERS AND PRE-SCHOOLERS

SARAH OCKWELL-SMITH
AUTHOR OF BABYCALM AND TODDLERCALM

piatkus

For my children,
Mummy is looking forward to waking you up at 6am
every day when you are all teenagers.

PIATKUS

First published in Great Britain in 2015 by Piatkus

5 7 9 10 8 6

A CIP catalogue record for this book
is available from the British Library.

ISBN 978-0-349-40520-9

Illustrations by Rodney Paull
Typeset in Stone Serif by M Rules
Printed and bound in Great Britain by
Clays Ltd, St Ives plc

Papers used by Piatkus are from well-managed forests
and other responsible sources.

MIX
Paper from
responsible sources
FSC
www.fsc.org   FSC® C104740

Piatkus
An imprint of
Little, Brown Book Group
100 Victoria Embankment
London EC4Y 0DY

An Hachette UK Company
www.hachette.co.uk

www.piatkus.co.uk

About the author

Sarah Ockwell-Smith is a mother of four who initially studied psychology at university. She has a BSc in Psychology and worked for several years in pharmaceutical research and development. Following the birth of her first child, Sarah retrained as a paediatric homeopath, HypnoBirthing antenatal teacher, and birth and postnatal doula. She has also undertaken training in baby massage, hypnotherapy and psychotherapy.

Sarah specialises in gentle parenting methods and has worked with over a thousand parents, helping them to settle into life as a new family and to cope with the challenges of raising their children from birth to school age. She blogs at www.sarahockwell-smith.com, writes for www.gentleparenting.co.uk and is the founder of BabyCalm™ (www.babycalm.co.uk) and ToddlerCalm™ (www.toddlercalm.co.uk), organisations offering parenting classes for those with babies and toddlers from birth to age three.

Contents

Acknowledgements

I would like to express my gratitude to all of the parents who have allowed me to publish their letters in this book. Their stories really help to bring my suggestions to life and without them this book would be hugely lacking.

A big thank-you to my agent Eve and her able assistant Jack, at Eve White Literary Agency, for their help and direction; and to Anne and Jillian at Piatkus, for continually making sense of what I am trying to say.

As ever, I am indebted to my family; to my husband and my children for their patience and pride in my work. I couldn't do it without you.

Lastly, thank you to you, the reader, for choosing to read my book over the myriad of other baby and child sleep books on the market. What an honour that is. I hope you enjoy *The Gentle Sleep Book* and that it helps you to get a little more sleep.

Foreword

'How is your baby sleeping?' It is the question all new parents face from family and strangers alike, and if the answer is anything less than 'It's wonderful! She's sleeping 12 hours a night', parents are treated to countless suggestions as to how they can 'improve' the situation.

We are a society obsessed with sleep. The amount your child sleeps is the yardstick by which other parents judge not only your parenting skills but also your child's development. In the eyes of many, failing to sleep 'well' within the appropriate time frame will ensure your child faces a bleak future from which he will never recover – and it will all be your fault. *Or so they say.*

In my own work, sleep issues make up approximately 90 per cent of the concerns or questions parents have. Even parents who admit that their sleep situation works well for them can reach the point where they start to wonder if they are doing something 'wrong' because their child isn't sleeping like they are 'supposed' to. In fact, the vast majority of questions about sleep focus on behaviours that the parents worry is 'bad' or will lead their child down the dreaded path towards never sleeping well.

For me, as someone who is trying to help these families, what is perhaps most frustrating is that, from a biological point of view, their child's behaviour is *entirely normal*.

Yes, normal. We may not realise it, but so much of what we have been led to believe is 'bad' or will damage our child's chances of sleeping – such as nursing to sleep, co-sleeping, or not having a set schedule for sleep – are not new inventions. Historically, children, particularly babies, did not have regimented sleep. They slept when they were tired, were often nursed to sleep, and slept close to their mother (facilitating breastfeeding at night and during the day). They 'learned' to sleep as adults did, which, contrary to what today's ideals dictate, was not throughout the night. As Sarah points out in the chapter on the history of sleep, adults sleeping through the night is a relatively new development that was partly brought about by the demands of the industrial revolution. It begs the question: are our expectations of children's sleep based more on cultural norms than their natural sleep patterns?

Much of what has been circulated in the parenting world on child sleep seems to be founded on parental convenience, rather than biology or science, and it's about time that changed. For example, if we think of the twelve-hour stretch at night as being a 'good' sleep or the 'right' amount of sleep, infant sleep is often rife with 'mistakes'. Their night wakings alone would have them failing the sleeping 'test', and the crying that often accompanies it would put them at the bottom of the class. However, if we think of that twelve-hour stretch as being a culturally dictated ideal, then we can start to look more sympathetically at what we might previously have considered 'failings' in our infants' sleep. In this book, Sarah Ockwell-Smith does a fantastic job of clarifying the research, pointing out the myths we have taken as fact, and the biological realities for our little ones.

For some of you, understanding what is happening with your child and her sleep will provide comfort and reassurance when things seem hard. For others, however, this won't be enough because the sleep deprivation you feel is so visceral that *something* has to be done. As Sarah rightfully points out, we have hit a false dichotomy in how we speak of infant sleep: in an effort to move away from the harsher forms of sleep training, we often see the only alternative as waiting it out when, in fact, is it not the only avenue open to us. There *are* gentle alternatives, yet we must beware the wolf in sheep's clothing. Many methods that claim to be gentle are anything but.

You need not fear the appearance of any wolf in the recommendations herein. You won't find one-size-fits-all solutions – and nor should you, given they don't acknowledge the unique needs of different children – but you will find advice and tips to help you reach a place of biologically normal, *good enough* sleep for everyone.

This book could not come at a better time. A recent survey in a popular parents' magazine found that 50 per cent of parents reported using the cry-it-out method with their babies. That's half of our children growing up with the expectation that nighttime is a time when their needs, fears and feelings are not valid or worthy of a response. That's half of parents believing that they don't have an alternative or that they have to do this to maintain sanity or keep their child from a worse fate. It's unfair to everyone involved.

As with her previous books, *BabyCalm* and *ToddlerCalm*, Sarah tackles the subjects of parental sleep deprivation, sleep guidance and the parent–child relationship with empathy, clarity and kindness. She also brings in the voices of many other parents who have 'been there and done that' so you need not feel like you're an island surrounded by water when it comes to your child's sleep. You won't find anything that tries to shame you or make you feel bad for steps already taken. Instead, you will feel heard and understood and given hope that your child's sleep need not cause the unraveling of your mind or your relationship with your child. I believe this book can bring you the peace and rest you need, while respecting the needs and feelings of your child, therefore helping you build a better and stronger relationship. After all, isn't that what all parenting advice should offer?

Sweet dreams,
Tracy Cassels, M.A., Ph.D. Candidate Founder,
EvolutionaryParenting.com

Introduction

Sleeping through the night

These four small words have an enormous impact on any parent of young children, especially when phrased in a question beginning with 'Are they . . .', and ending in 'yet?'. It's even worse when they are uttered by friends whose perfect child sleeps for twelve hours straight every night and has done since he was six weeks old. There's no doubt about it, child sleep – or the lack of – can leave even the most confident of parents feeling like a failure.

The first five years of parenting are filled with worries and pre-occupations, but, for the vast majority, none of them is as pressing as the lack of sleep. Research shows that almost one-third of all parents of babies and small children consider their child's sleep 'problematic'.[1] I think that figure is rather conservative: my experience of working with parents would suggest it is as high as two-thirds, if not more.

I can't say I remember those early sleep-deprived years with my own four children well, even though it wasn't that long ago. Nature has a funny way of erasing the exhaustion and trauma from our memories. My memories are almost all happy ones imbued with feelings of pride, peace, contentment and happiness.

When I look back now, I remember the sweet scent of baby breath being softly exhaled as I sat watching them sleep soundly; my husband carrying sleeping toddlers in from the car, hair damp on one side of their head, while they still clutched a beloved soft toy; and trying to change them into their pyjamas before they woke. I remember my pre-schoolers falling asleep on the sofa while waiting for me to prepare their lunch, tired from the excitement of their morning's activities.

One day I am sure your memories will be positive too, and the exhaustion and desperation of your non-sleeping child will be replaced with something altogether happier. Right now though, I know that is not the case and no matter how many of your friends tell you 'it won't last forever', such comments don't help. When I was a sleep-deprived parent what I really needed was a combination of reassurance, reliable information and easy-to-follow advice. This is exactly what I hope to provide in this book.

As a sleep-deprived parent, I remember searching for the Holy Grail of sleep advice – evidence-based and gentle, but effective. Some advice suggested I should just 'wait it out' and one day my child would claim their 'I slept through the night' medal. Understandably, for most parents, this is neither practical nor feasible. We live in a world where parents are expected to do more than just parent; many need to go out to work, often for long hours. They often have to parent without a close support network around them. There is no denying that parenting today is incredibly stressful; in some ways perhaps more so than for any generation before. Often the demands of modern-day parenting mean that just 'waiting it out' can be to the detriment of the child as well as the adult. Having exhausted, wrung out, angry, desperate and depressed parents cannot be in the best interests of any child.

Somewhere there must be a happy medium. You need reliable information and advice that empowers you to make the right decisions for your family's unique situation while considering everybody's needs. This is exactly the gap I hope to fill with this book, because your child isn't the only one whose feelings matter; yours do too. The real goal of parenting is to tread a carefully balanced line where everybody's needs are considered equally. Throughout this book I endeavour to treat parents and their children as a team. Some child sleep experts focus on pitting parent against child, portraying sleep as a battle that is won by one or the other. Yet if a parent 'wins' the sleep battle, that leaves the child the 'loser', with the battle scars to show for it; something no parent wants for their child.

One of the best ways to empower parents struggling with their child's sleep is to provide information that helps them to understand their child's behaviour. Some sleep experts might suggest that there is a 'secret' to sleep success, but I believe that there is no such thing. If there was it surely wouldn't be a secret, would it? Parents around the world would be shouting it from the rooftops. The trouble is, when you are sleep deprived and unable to think straight, these claims can seem incredibly appealing.

The vast majority of parents turn to the internet for help with their child's sleep. As it becomes more and more easy to publish online, it follows that the chance of reading incorrect and sometimes even dangerous information increases. It is really important to read sleep-related articles on the internet (and in magazines for that matter) with a hefty degree of scepticism. As paediatrician and SIDS (sudden infant death syndrome) expert Dr Rachel Moon said in her research, conducted in 2012: 'It is important for health care providers to realize the extent to which parents may turn to the internet for information about infant sleep safety and then act on that advice, regardless of the reliability of the source.' Dr Moon found that 72 per cent of parents believed that information regarding health issues on the internet was trustworthy, with 70 per cent saying they had used information found on the internet in an attempt to help their child's sleep. Dr Moon's study, of 1,300 websites offering child sleep information, found that 28 per cent contained inaccurate information.[2] More alarmingly, even government websites contained many errors, with 20 per cent of the sleep information presented being inaccurate.

Inaccurate sleep advice is not just found on the internet and in books and magazines. Some health professionals, including GPs and health visitors, give inaccurate advice, particularly on sleep training, bedsharing, weaning and breastfeeding. You would be forgiven for thinking that information from health professionals must be factually correct and in your child's best interests, but what many parents don't realise is how little training professionals receive on the subject of paediatric sleep and related psychology. Moreover, this information is rarely updated with the latest research findings and is often centred on the health professional's personal opinions and own parenting experiences, which are very often anything but evidence-based.

While writing this book I asked hundreds of parents for their answers to the question, 'What is the most important thing that you have learnt about child sleep?' Interestingly, many commented on the reliability or otherwise of common sleep advice. Here are a few of their comments:

> Ninety-five per cent of what new parents are told about the subject is false. All children are different, and parents are better off when they don't worry about anything concerning the phrase 'sleeping through the night'.

> Throw out the rulebook and guidelines!

> Waking during the night is biologically normal and healthy.

> Understand that your child doesn't understand the rules and just desperately needs your love.

Trust your intuition at all times, even when you're a first-time mum: you know your child best, so do what feels right.

In this book I hope to treat you with the respect that you and your child deserve. I do not endorse any methods that will leave you or your child feeling alone or distressed. Perhaps most importantly, I have backed up as much information as possible with scientific research findings. If you are interested in learning more about these you will find the references at the back of the book.

I never fail to be surprised at the powerful effect of giving parents the facts about 'normal' baby and child sleep. Some simple science and statistics can transform a parent's opinion of their child's sleep. It can help to normalise their child's behaviour, which can allay any concerns and guilt parents may be feeling for perhaps 'not being good enough' or worrying that they did something wrong. For this reason I devote the whole of the first chapter of this book to the science of child sleep, as it seems an obvious place to start. Reading this chapter will help you to feel more positive straight away. It certainly had a profound impact on these mothers:

Learning that they are not all sleeping through the night until well after two years old. What a relief that was!

Remember your child is not broken; you are not doing it wrong, it's just 'normal'.

It's perfectly normal not to sleep through the night until the toddler years or beyond. I would have been so stressed out by now if I hadn't discovered this.

Definitely the best thing I learnt about child sleep was knowing about brain development!

> Knowing that frequent waking during the night is totally normal for a baby/toddler really helped. It is still hard at times, but just that knowledge makes a big difference.

Also, bear in mind that when it comes to child sleep 'normal' is a very wide category. I'm sure you've seen charts listing the amount of hours a day that a baby, toddler or pre-schooler should sleep. It may surprise you to learn that until the end of 2013 these were based almost entirely on opinion and guess-work. It is only very recently that scientists have begun to study the sleep patterns of childhood in any great detail. I will outline the most up-to-date scientific research findings in Chapter 1, but it is important to remember that these numbers are a guide and an average. There will always be children who need more or less sleep, longer or shorter naps. Just because your child isn't 'average' doesn't mean anything is wrong. This is why it is so important to take an individualised approach to child sleep, because what works for one family may not work for another.

In Chapter 2 I look at the history of sleep, how our sleeping patterns have changed through the centuries and, crucially, how modern life has impacted on our sleep. One concept that I will examine is that of the primitive infant in a modern world. Babies don't know that they have been born in the twenty-first century. They don't know that they should behave differently to babies born in the sixteenth century, yet as adults our lives couldn't be more different. The primal needs of babies and young children are very often at odds with the modern needs of today's parents, which makes parenting harder for all. As ever, the answer lies in providing information and in trying to balance the needs of everyone involved.

On a similar theme, in Chapter 3 I look at the anthropology of sleep – the study of sleep around the world. I look at how parents from different cultures handle bedtime and naps, how their expectations and sleep arrangements may differ and if they share the same problems with their children's sleep as parents in the West. I will go on to consider what can be learnt from the parenting practices of other cultures.

Another hot topic at the moment is the impact of diet on child sleep. Do breastfed and formula-fed babies sleep differently? Does introducing a bottle or a 'dream-feed' help a baby to sleep through the night? Does weaning onto solids encourage longer stretches of sleep? Does your toddler's tiny appetite impact on his sleep? Could what your four-year-old eats during the day have an impact on how she sleeps at night? Are there any foods that aid sleep? Are there any that should be avoided? I examine these issues and more in Chapter 4. Chapter 5 looks at the problems associated with using modern sleep-training techniques.

I am well aware that while knowledge is hugely empowering, you haven't bought this book simply for background information. You are looking for practical suggestions to help your family have more peaceful days and quieter nights. This is the purpose of 'BEDTIME', which I introduce in Chapter 6. This acronym covers what I believe to be the seven most important general points to think about and implement when trying to encourage your child to sleep more easily. They can be applied to all families and to children of all ages, from newborn to age five and beyond.

In the remainder of the book I take you through sleep information that is specific to your child's age, from birth to the age of five. Sleep needs and biology change dramatically over the first five years of life and the approach with a tiny baby is very different to one you may take with a four-year-old. Each chapter features parents and children I have worked with, who have kindly agreed to share their stories. These case studies will help you to understand the underlying reasons for each family's struggles, and how they applied some of the points in my BEDTIME strategy in order to come up with a unique plan for their child.

The final chapter provides the understanding and tools you need to create your own unique sleep plan for your child, and bring peace back to your family.

A note on how to use this book

I have written the first six chapters of this book to apply to all parents, no matter how old your child is or what their sleep problem may be. Chapters 7 to 12 give specific advice, based upon the age of the child. In Chapter 13 I sum up the issues covered in the rest of the book and help you to formulate a plan for your own family. Ideally, you should read chapters 1 to 6 first, before moving on to the age-specific advice: if read in this way, the tips contained in chapters 7 to 12 make a lot more sense. I appreciate, however, that some people may be desperate for practical tips that they can use immediately. Chapters 7 to 12 are relatively free-standing, if you need something to try right now. Please do go back and read chapters 1 to 6, though, when you have time. Obviously, as your child grows, you can dip back into the chapter that is specific to your child's age without having to re-read the whole book.

Chapter 1

Understanding normal sleep physiology

How much do you know about the normal physiology of child sleep? I didn't know very much when I was a new parent, and I didn't even think to research it. I spent hours researching ways in which to encourage my child to sleep for longer, go to bed earlier and wake later, but I never once thought to pick up one of the dusty old psychobiology books I had on my shelf and learn more about the basics of sleep. None of the parenting magazines I read or websites I visited looked at sleep in this way either; they all jumped straight into 'fixing problems'. How, though, do you know if your child has a problem if you don't know what is normal? It strikes me that many sleep-related articles start at 'point 2' (fixing the problem) and completely bypass 'point 1' (*is* there actually a problem?).

I firmly believe that the biology of sleep should be taught to all parents. We spend so long learning about labour and childbirth but very little time learning about what happens *after* the baby is born. If we do, usually all our efforts are focused on nappy changing, feeding and bathing, but isn't sleep as important? It would be useful if all parents also took a class covering the basics of sleep for the first few years of life: it would be invaluable if they were taught what to expect realistically at each age and given an explanation of why their child behaved in a certain way related to sleep. I have worked with numerous families who see an astounding difference once they have a good grasp of some basic sleep biology. That is why this chapter is devoted to exactly that.

Sleep is as vital to our survival as food and water, but most people know far more about the latter two topics. The more you can educate yourself on the science of sleep the more able you are to help yourself and your children in your own unique family situation.

So, what happens when we close our eyes and drift off to sleep? Sleep is essentially a chemically controlled process. That is not to say it isn't affected by external influences, it is, and I'll talk about those throughout this book, but the basic building blocks of sleep are chemical ones. At the base of your brain is a section called the brainstem, which connects your brain and spinal cord. The brainstem is often referred to as the 'primitive' or 'reptilian' part of the brain as it resembles the unsophisticated, primitive brain of a reptile. The brainstem, along with a section of the brain called the hypothalamus, is responsible for what is known as 'homoeostasis', or basic life support functions, such as breathing, temperature regulation, eating and, importantly here, sleeping.

Circadian rhythms and melatonin

The brainstem and hypothalamus contain neurons, special cells that transmit nerve impulses. Neurons produce neurotransmitters, chemical messengers that carry the impulses between cells.

These neurons and chemicals can make us feel sleepy or awake and do so over a period of twenty-four hours. This recurring twenty-four-hour sleep/wake cycle is more commonly referred to as a circadian rhythm. The word 'circadian' derives from the Latin phrase *'circa dies'*, which means 'around a day'.

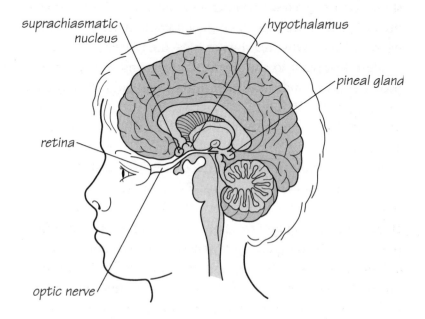

Our circadian rhythms are controlled by the hypothalamus, or, more specifically, a snappily named, pinhead-sized part of the hypothalamus called the suprachiasmatic nucleus (or SCN for short). The SCN is full of thousands of neurons and is situated at the back of the eyes close to the optic nerves. There is a special reason it is situated in this area: when light hits the back of our eyes (a part known as the retina) the light-sensitive photoreceptors transmit a signal down the optic nerves to the SCN. The SCN then transmits signals to other parts of our brain, the most significant being the pineal gland, which looks like a mini pine cone, hence the name.

The pineal gland is one of the most important areas to look at when it comes to sleep, as it responds to the presence of light by inhibiting the production of melatonin. Melatonin is known to many as 'the hormone of sleep' and levels naturally rise after darkness (due to the process described above), making us feel sleepy. As well as affecting the secretion of melatonin, the SCN also regulates other functions linked to our circadian rhythms, such as body temperature and the production of urine, both of which are lowered at night. When the sun rises in the morning, the light exposure causes the SCN to transmit signals to raise body temperature and secrete the hormone cortisol (and inhibit melatonin), which helps us to feel alert.

The development of circadian rhythms

The most pertinent point to understand with regard to circadian rhythms and child sleep is that they take time to develop. Babies are not born with circadian rhythms, although, while in utero, melatonin does pass into the body via the umbilical cord and the mother's body and babies exhibit similar sleep/wake patterns to their mother.[1] Obviously this transfusion of sleep hormones ceases after birth and babies are left without any circadian rhythms of their own. This explains why newborns sleep sporadically throughout the day and night. A newborn baby has no concept of night and day; their bodies are as incapable of telling the difference between night and day as they are of telling the time from a clock. The development of circadian rhythms is purely biological and, like many developmental milestones that happen throughout childhood, it cannot be rushed. A baby's circadian rhythms will mature when the neurobiological processes in the baby's brain are complete, so there is little parents can do but wait for this to happen. Some baby experts advocate the use of blackout blinds, getting babies changed at night and keeping communication to a minimum at night-time in the hope of 'teaching baby night from day'. This only serves to give parents something to do so that they feel they are helping.

In the last twenty years many scientists have researched the development of circadian rhythms and have concluded that sleep-related circadian rhythms do not begin to emerge until the eighth week after birth.[2] Further research indicates that circadian rhythms are not well established until babies are around four months of age.[3] It is therefore around this age that you can expect a baby's sleep patterns to show some response to the difference between night and day.

Early waking and circadian rhythms

I am often asked for help with the 'problem' of early waking. If we look at this in the context of circadian rhythms, it is obvious that, for young children, waking at the crack of dawn is a normal biological response to light. In fact, it may be that our adult circadian rhythms are dulled by our modern lifestyle and we are the ones with the problem.

That said, even if early waking is not a problem in the strictest sense of the word, the fact remains that for lots of parents it *is* a challenge. The only solution to early waking is to adjust your own lifestyle to better cope with your child's early waking, and to ensure their safety in the morning, if they wake before you. If the child is old enough, you can consider ways to keep her occupied for a little time in the morning so that you can get a little more sleep, but that really is as good as it gets.

What happens during sleep?

The phrase 'sleep through the night' is very misleading. In reality, nobody sleeps through the night: we all move through different levels of sleep and often wake, sometimes so briefly we have no memory of it the next morning; at other times our nocturnal wakings are obvious and we have trouble returning to sleep. Understanding that nobody simply goes to sleep at night and wakes in the morning is vital when it comes to understanding child sleep.

So what does a night's sleep look like? Sleep is predominantly divided into two types, rapid eye movement (REM) and non-rapid eye movement (NREM), but the length of these cycles and the order in which they occur varies hugely with age.

REM (active) sleep

In REM (or active) sleep our muscles are effectively paralysed, but our eyes move rapidly underneath our closed eyelids, hence the name. In contrast to this muscle paralysis, the neurons in our brain are incredibly active; indeed scientists sometimes refer to REM as 'paradoxical sleep' because of this strange contrast. REM is also the stage of sleep where vivid dreams occur. REM sleep is said to be especially important to the developing brain in babies and young children, with researchers hypothesising that the increased neural stimulation that happens during this stage is necessary in order to create new neural connections in the developing brain.[4]

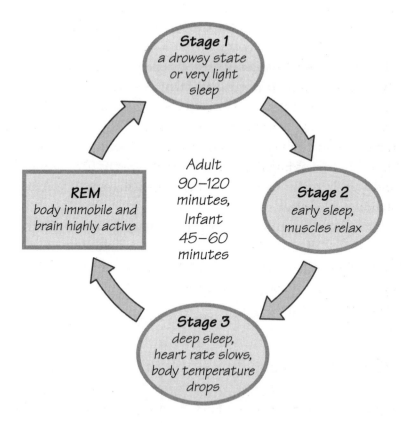

NREM (quiet) sleep

NREM (or quiet) sleep is further sub-divided. These stages are:

N1: A very light sleep or a deep level of drowsiness and relaxation. During this stage the eyes are usually closed, but it is very easy to wake fully.

N2: This is the early stage of sleep. Muscles start to relax, the heart rate begins to slow and body temperature begins to drop.

N3: A deeper level of sleep, it is much harder to awaken during this phase. The body relaxes more, with further reductions in body temperature and heart rate. The earlier part of this phase of sleep is where sleepwalking and sleeptalking most commonly occur. The latter end of this phase of sleep is where dreaming, nightmares, night terrors and bed-wetting are most likely to occur.

The difference in sleep cycles by age

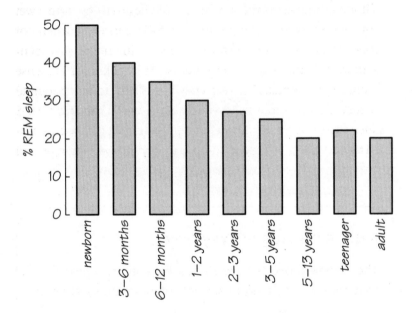

Newborns to age three months

In the first few months of life, a baby's sleep looks very different to that of an adult. At this age a baby not only lacks the hormonal regulators of sleep provided by circadian rhythms but their sleep cycles are also roughly half the length of an adult's, at around forty to forty-five minutes long. In contrast to an adult, whose sleep comprises around 20 per cent REM, young babies spend a huge 50 per cent of their sleep in the REM phase.

Babies begin their sleep cycle with REM, or active, sleep, where they stay for around twenty minutes. During this time they can be easily awoken. The final twenty minutes of a young baby's sleep cycle is spent in NREM, or quiet, sleep. This stage of sleep is deeper and the baby is less likely to wake in response to stimulation. At the end of this cycle the baby may wake entirely, or, if nothing alerts them, they may begin a new forty-minute cycle. You can see here that, effectively, young babies may wake every twenty minutes if something alerts them, which could be anything from a wet nappy, feeling cold or feeling hungry to feeling insecure when not in your arms (which isn't surprising considering he has just spent nine months being held inside a uterus). This makes perfect sense in evolutionary terms, as it keeps newborns alert to any potential predators or harm and is believed to help protect a baby from SIDS (sudden infant death syndrome), but for parents it can be exhausting. The best thing to keep in mind is that things will change, and fairly quickly, as your baby's sleep physiology matures.

A NOTE ON SIDS PREVENTION

The following points have all been scientifically proven to reduce a baby's risk of sudden infant death syndrome:

- Always place your baby to sleep on their back, never on their front.

- Do not smoke during pregnancy and do not let anyone smoke around your baby.

- Keep your baby in the same room as you for at least the first six months.

- Always place your baby to sleep on a firm surface and make sure you never fall asleep with them on a sofa.

- If you share a bed with your baby, make sure you follow safer bedsharing guidelines (see page 97).

- Do not allow your baby to overheat and do not use loose blankets, which may suffocate your baby.

- If you swaddle your baby, make sure you follow safer swaddling guidelines (see page 129).

- Breastfeed your baby exclusively for as long as you can, preferably until they are at least six months old.

Age three to six months

This period is a busy one for babies sleep-wise, as big changes happen. The first is the development of a circadian rhythm, which goes from almost non-existent at the beginning of this period to relatively sophisticated by the end. This means that at some point between three and six months your baby's body develops the ability to tell the difference between night and day, and hopefully they will begin to sleep more at night and less in the day.

In addition to the development of a body clock, the amount of REM sleep a baby experiences between three and six months drops to around 40 per cent. This means that they spend more time in the 'quiet' sleep state of NREM and, theoretically, awaken less to external stimuli, although their sleep cycle is still only around forty-five minutes long.

Age six to twelve months

By this stage, a baby's circadian rhythm is almost comparable to that of an adult and their sleep timings and body clock should be very much in line with that of their parents, albeit with more awakenings at night and naps during the day. REM sleep drops to around 35 per cent by this stage, meaning that 'quiet' NREM sleep makes up around two-thirds of your baby's sleep cycle. Although their sleep cycle is still only around fifty minutes long, still much shorter than that of an adult, the increased amount of NREM sleep means that, theoretically, they wake less than they did before six months of age. Often this is not the case though, due to the appearance of teething and, in some cases, separation anxiety (see Chapter 9 for more on this).

Age one to two years

By this stage the proportion of REM sleep has dropped to around 30 per cent and NREM (quiet) sleep stages are well established. The average sleep cycle lasts around sixty minutes and naps in the day are still common, although less so than in the first year. Biologically speaking, this means that a toddler's night-time sleep should be fairly comparable to that of an adult. Psychologically speaking, however, other issues come into play, which can mean that a toddler's sleep is anything but comparable to that of an adult's, and many parents report a regression in their child's sleep at this age.

Age two to three years

REM sleep now consists of around 27 per cent of the night's sleep. Daytime naps are still common; however, many children no longer need them towards the end of this time period. Sleep cycles are lengthening and this, combined with almost three-quarters of sleep being 'quiet' with well-defined NREM stages, means that, biologically, sleep is in line with that of an adult. Other issues have an effect, however, from the arrival of a new sibling, to starting pre-school and potty training. This means that although, biologically, a full night's sleep is possible, practical or psychological reasons often prevent it.

Age three to five years

REM now accounts for only 20–25 per cent of the sleep cycle, similar to that of an adult's sleep. The sleep cycle itself also lengthens and towards the end of this period is fairly comparable to that of an adult, at around seventy to ninety minutes. Daytime naps usually disappear by the end of this period, although for many this may be due more to environmental factors, such as starting school, rather than the child's innate needs. Despite sleep being biologically comparable to that of an adult at this age, many factors still prevent children from sleeping in the way parents would like them to. This is the peak age for the onset of night terrors, nightmares, sleepwalking and sleeptalking. Bed-wetting is also still common, affecting around 80 per cent of children at the younger end of this category and 20 per cent at the older end. Add to this the effects of starting school and it's hardly surprising that sleep problems are still common in this age range. Some research has indicated that 50 per cent of pre-schoolers wake regularly at night.[5] See Chapter 12 for more on this.

Genetics versus environment

No parenting book would be complete without a 'nature versus nurture' argument. It's not quite as simple as either/or when it comes to sleep, however. While we know that for the first five years of life a very large proportion of sleep behaviour is due entirely to the child's biology and genetic make-up, there is no denying that external influences come into play too.

Research looking at the sleeping behaviour of twins has found that night-time sleep had at least a 50 per cent genetic basis; however, nap times in the day are influenced far more by environmental factors. The researchers commented that 'early childhood daytime sleep duration could be influenced by environmental settings, while the variance in consolidated night-time sleep duration is impacted mostly by genetic factors'.[6] The environmental effect on naps seems to peak at around the age of two, where it has been found to have as much as a 79 per cent influence on the length of daytime naps taken by children. The environmental influence on naps, however, is far less when a child is younger: for instance, an eighteen-month-old is far more affected by biology, with the environment having only a 33 per cent influence upon the length of daytime naps. These findings are in line with the general thinking that babies and young toddlers are primarily governed by biological and developmental processes when it comes to sleep, while older toddlers' and pre-schoolers' sleep is much more affected by environmental and psychological factors.

How much sleep should children have?

I'm sure that you will have seen several tables indicating how many hours of daytime and night-time sleep your child *should* have at any given age. These tables are often presented as fact and can be the cause of great concern if you have a child who is sleeping significantly less (or more) than the average time for their age. Infuriatingly though, these guidelines are just that, guidelines, not rules, and for many children they simply do not apply. Perhaps more alarming, until very recently, these timings were not evidence-based but simply estimates of what professionals thought children should be doing. And of course that's often very different to what children actually do!

Another inconsistency prevalent in the field of paediatric sleep is the notion that our children are grossly sleep deprived and that this could spell doom and gloom for their future health and intelligence. Again, in most cases, this is simply not true. It is true that over the last century the amount our children sleep has declined, but more pertinent is the fact that for at least one hundred years our babies and children have not been getting the amount of sleep recommended. In other words, this 'new', well-publicised phenomenon of a gross lack of sleep in children is not new at all. I would argue that the recommendations are wrong, not our children's sleep patterns.

In 2012, a team of researchers from Australia surveyed over two hundred parents and carried out analysis of sleep recommendations dating from 1897 to 2009. Their aim was to compare the recommendations with the amount of time children actually slept. Professor of Health Sciences at the University of South Australia, Dr Tim Olds, commented, 'Never trust sleep experts. One child may function best on 7 hours, another on 11 hours.'[7] Dr Olds points out that there is no such thing as a norm for the amount of sleep a child needs as all children are different. He believes it is more important that our children get the amount of sleep required to meet their individual needs. This is something I strongly agree with, as do these mothers I spoke to during the course of writing this book.

Sleep is only a problem when it's a problem for me and my family, not when others tell me it's a problem.

Each child is an individual and what works for one may not work for another. My little boy needed lots of sleep, but my little girl seems to be allergic to it. Follow their cues and you won't go far wrong.

No matter what you do, he will sleep when he is ready, for the amount of time he needs, and that's OK.

Putting pressure on yourself or your child to do 'what is expected' only adds stress and makes you more tired emotionally.

What works for your family might not work for someone else's and vice versa.

It changes all the time! Just go with the flow. You'll drive yourself crazy trying to force a pattern that isn't there!

It's much easier to deal with if you just accept what is, rather than worrying about what you think should be.

It's completely down to the specific child.

In 2012, research conducted in England confirmed that the amount of sleep needed at various ages varies wildly. Analysing data from over 11,000 children, the researchers found that even for babies, sleep duration ranged widely from eleven to seventeen hours in a twenty-four-hour period. This variation narrowed as the children got older but there was still a variation of two and a half hours per day for the older children.[8]

Research published in 2014 attempted, for the first time ever, to provide accurate norms for child sleep needs and expectations from birth to age nine years, based upon evidence not opinion. A team of researchers from Australia studied reports of the sleep patterns of 10,000 children, including both naps and night-time sleep. A huge variability in sleep patterns was found at all ages, from bedtime, to wake time, nap time and overall sleep duration. The study's lead researcher, Dr Anna Price, said, 'Whether a child is getting enough sleep or how much sleep a child needs is a major concern to many parents. In this study we found there is a wide range in "normal" child sleep from four months to nine years old.'[9]

The main findings of this research are summarised in the table below:

Age of child	Total sleep per 24 hrs (in hours)	Total nap duration (in hours)	Total night wakings (in minutes)	Average wake time	Average bedtime
4–6 months	14	3	26.9	7:30	20:00
7–9 months	13.6	2.7	20.3	7:15	20:00
10–12 months	13.4	2.5	14.3	7:00	20:00
13–15 months	13.4	2.4	11.7	7:00	20:00
2 years	11.9	1	4.4	7:15	20:15
3 years	11.7	0.8	3.8	7:15	20:15
4 years	11.2	0.3	2.8	7:15	20:30
5 years	10.5	0.2	2.1	7:15	20:30

Two findings of this research stand out for me. First, how most current child sleep guidelines vastly overestimate the amount of sleep needed for each age group. For instance, the NHS website recommends that two-year-olds should have a total of thirteen hours' sleep in twenty-four hours. The findings of the Australian study, however, indicate that the two-year-olds in their research were only sleeping for a total of eleven hours and fifty-four minutes. Similarly, the NHS website recommends that six-month-olds should nap for four hours every day, when the Australian research found that they napped for only three. Almost every recommendation on the NHS website, for both total sleep duration and nap duration, is higher than the Australian research found. If you are a parent whose child is sleeping less than the recommendations on the NHS website I can appreciate how stressful and worrying this may be, yet it is highly likely that your child's sleep is normal. Many scientists and sleep specialists now highlight how much sleep duration varies and how important it is to recognise a child's sleep needs as individual. Clearly this message has not filtered through to the media.

The second point that really stands out for me in the Australian research is the relatively late average bedtimes, particularly for toddlers. I am quite often contacted by parents wanting help to get their toddler or pre-schooler to bed at night. When I ask what time they are putting their child to bed they often reply 7pm or 7.30pm. Looking at the table you can see that this is an hour earlier than the average toddler or pre-schooler sleeps. I will examine this idea of a later bedtime, and how it may actually help everyone to get more sleep, in more depth in the next chapter and in chapters 11 to 13.

Common sleep disorders in early childhood

Sleep apnoea and snoring

Sleep apnoea and snoring both fall under the label of 'sleep disordered breathing', but they are very different. Sleep apnoea occurs when a child stops breathing for a short amount of time, say for ten seconds or more. Sleep apnoea affects between 0.7 and 1.8 per cent of all children under sixteen. An article in the *British Medical Journal* (*BMJ*) describes sleep apnoea as 'a disorder of breathing during sleep that is characterised by prolonged partial upper airway obstruction and/or intermittent complete obstruction that adversely affects ventilation during sleep and disrupts normal sleep patterns'.[10] This means that when air is inhaled during sleep, a time when muscles are naturally relaxed, a child's airway occasionally falls in on itself, making it harder to breathe. The body senses that there is a problem and the child will then often struggle to breathe, which may temporarily exacerbate the issue. Ultimately, the child will reach a level of arousal that allows them to clear their airway and go back to sleep. It is unlikely that the child will remember this when they wake in the morning. Understandably, this pattern can not only negatively impact the child's sleep patterns, but it can also be incredibly stressful for parents to witness.

Sleep apnoea in children is commonly caused by an obstruction in the child's airways, such as enlarged tonsils or adenoids (or both), or a structural abnormality in the child's palate or shape of the head or neck. Allergies can play a role, too. Sleep apnoea can have complications so it is important that you speak to your GP if you think your child may be affected and ask for a referral to a paediatric ear, nose and throat (ENT) specialist.

The same *BMJ* article describes snoring as 'noisy breathing caused by turbulent airflow', which simply refers to noise made during breathing while asleep. Snoring occurs in approximately 12 per cent of all children under sixteen on any given night, but most children snore at some point, particularly during the deepest phase of NREM sleep. Persistent snoring in children could be a sign of enlarged tonsils or adenoids, as with sleep apnoea. Again, if you are concerned, visit your GP.

Nightmares

Nightmares are incredibly common during childhood, with most children suffering at some point, although they are more common in girls than boys. Nightmares are a form of vivid dream and, as such, they occur in REM sleep. They often start at around two years of age and reach a peak between the ages of three and six. Children experiencing a nightmare are very likely to wake up and need your help to calm them and help them return to sleep. Children will often remember the theme of their nightmares and can describe them in great detail. Nightmares commonly occur towards the end of a night's sleep, as morning approaches, and are linked to anxiety, witnessing traumatic events and, most commonly, watching scary television programmes.

The most obvious course of action is to try to work out the cause and, if possible, remove it from the child's life, as well as comforting them when they wake. I have always allowed my children into my bed after they have woken from a nightmare, as I feel it's a time when they need my reassurance and constant physical presence the most. You could also read them stories that talk about their fears, in the hope of lessening them through the safe medium of storytelling (see page 282 for some suggestions). However you respond, it is important to realise that the child's fears are very real to them, so you must respect this. Don't be tempted to say something like 'Don't be silly, there's no such thing as monsters', as this dismisses your child's fears and will do little to help him. Instead, respond with something along the lines of 'Oh, monsters can be scary can't they? What does your one look like? What do you think we can do to frighten it away?'

Research conducted at the University of Tel Aviv in 2012 found that children who experienced nightmares had difficulty separating fantasy from reality, something that is heightened the younger the child is. The lead researcher, Professor Sadeh, said, 'We send children mixed signals by telling them that monsters aren't real while we tell them stories about the tooth fairy ... Simply telling a child that their fear isn't realistic doesn't solve the problem.' Instead, he suggests using the imagination of the child in order to reduce their fears: for example, help the child to write a letter to the monster asking for a truce and read them bedtime stories about monsters and nightmares that turn out not to be so scary after all. Professor Sadeh found that allowing the child to transfer their fear and worry onto a stuffed toy, which they then care for and help not to be so afraid, can help significantly, too.[11]

When my own children were suffering from nightmares I took a more creative approach by choosing a Native American dream catcher with them, and explain how they 'catch' bad dreams but let the good ones through, before hanging it in their room. I also made 'monster spray' (which was nothing more than water, food dye and glitter in a clear plastic spray bottle) and in the evenings we made a big fuss of going on an elaborate 'monster hunt' in their room, with the child in charge of spraying all of the dark corners and under the bed with the magic spray, which repels monsters. I left the monster spray on their bedside table for them to use in the night if they ever felt like they needed it. It certainly seemed to work.

Night terrors

Night terrors are very different to nightmares and are relatively rare, affecting around 3 per cent of children.[12] They occur during the last stages of NREM sleep, which means that affected children are very difficult to arouse during an episode and they will have no memory of the night terror when they wake. During a night terror a child can appear to be awake, often with their eyes open, thrashing around, hitting out and even talking, but they are very much asleep. Night terrors can last anything from a minute or two up to fifteen minutes and most commonly appear in the earlier part of the night, before midnight. However, despite the name, they can also occur during daytime naps. The most common time of onset is around three years of age, although they can start earlier and, in contrast to nightmares, tend to affect more boys than girls.

Night terrors can be incredibly distressing for parents, but take heart from the fact that your child will have no memory of the events. The most important response is to ensure that your child is safe and cannot hurt himself, then try to calm him – but don't be surprised if this has little effect, as often it is a case of letting the terror run its course. Research by consultant psychiatrist Professor Bryan Lask, carried out at Great Ormond Street Hospital in London, may provide hope for parents of children suffering from night terrors. Professor Lask suggests that parents make a note of the time that their child's night terrors occur for five nights in a row. If there is a pattern to the child's night terrors, he suggests waking the child around ten to fifteen minutes before the night terror usually starts and keeping them awake for five minutes, before allowing them to return to sleep. The process should be repeated each evening until the terrors are extinguished, which in his research was less than a week for all cases.[13]

There is no single known cause of night terrors, but there

does appear to be a genetic link, as they seem to run in families. Some suggest that night terrors are more common if children are experiencing a period of stress or are overtired, whereas others say this is not the case. Most children simply grow out of night terrors.

Sleepwalking

Sleepwalking (also known as somnambulism) is fairly common, and it is thought that up to a third of all children will sleepwalk at some point, with the most common age of onset being between three and seven. Nobody is really sure what the cause of sleepwalking is, but there seems to be a genetic link and if you sleepwalk then your child is more likely to do so.

Despite the name, some children don't actually walk around when sleepwalking; some may just sit up in their bed. In most cases, the child's eyes will be open, although it tends to be obvious that they are not awake as they will appear to look straight through you. Episodes of sleepwalking occur during the deepest phase of NREM sleep and tend to last for between one and ten minutes. At the end of the episode most children will return to bed and seem to fall back to sleep, although they have never really been awake in the first place. They are unlikely to remember their sleepwalking in the morning.

Most children will grow out of sleepwalking naturally and there isn't any specific treatment beyond making sure that your child is safe. If your child is a sleepwalker it is better not to use a mid-sleeper (a bed with drawers or a play area underneath), bunk or cabin bed, and you might consider fitting a stair-gate at the top of the stairs to make sure they do not fall down them when on their travels. As alarming as it may be to witness your child sleepwalking, it is very common and nothing to worry about once you have ensured your child's safety.

Sleeptalking

Sleeptalking (also known as somniloquy) is similar to sleep-walking in that it is fairly common and nothing to be alarmed by. Up to 50 per cent of children talk in their sleep at some point: onset is usually between three and seven years. Each episode can last anything from just a few seconds up to around a minute or more and, as with sleepwalking, it occurs in the deepest phase of NREM sleep. Sometimes the child will appear to talk complete nonsense; other times they can be very eloquent and may appear to be holding a conversation with you. Sleeptalking appears to run in families and affects boys and girls equally.

There is no treatment for sleeptalking so the aim is to keep the disruption to the rest of the family to a minimum, for instance avoid siblings sharing the same room if one is a sleeptalker. Children usually grow out of sleeptalking, although 10 per cent of adults still talk in their sleep.

Bed-wetting

Bed-wetting (or enuresis) is incredibly common and a natural part of childhood in most cases. It is perfectly normal for children to sleep in nappies at night until they are at school, sometimes right up to seven years of age, although in our society there does seem to be a bit of a fixation on children being 'dry at night' very early on. Estimates of the incidence of bed-wetting indicate that around 10 per cent of two-year-olds will be reliably dry at night, rising to 20 per cent at age three, 55 per cent at age four and around 80 per cent at age five.[14] This means that around a quarter of all reception children will still wet the bed with some regularity. Bed-wetting is slightly more common in boys than girls. Most medical professionals do not consider bed-wetting a problem until seven years of age.

In most cases, bed-wetting is due to an immature bladder that is not yet large enough to accommodate the amount of urine produced. It can also affect children who sleep very deeply and therefore do not wake up in response to the body's urge to urinate. Sometimes bed-wetting can be in response to an overactive bladder or constipation. It can also be due to anxiety and other emotional causes, though this tends to affect older children more. Like sleepwalking and talking and night terrors, bed-wetting most commonly occurs in the deepest phase of NREM sleep.

Most importantly, do not make bed-wetting a big issue so that it upsets or embarrasses your child. Reassure them that 'it's OK; it's really common to wet the bed when you're little as your body is still learning to control itself'. Never punish a child for wetting the bed, however tired or angry you are at having to deal with yet another change of sheets at 2am.

A useful trick is to make up the child's bed twice, with a waterproof protector on top of the mattress, a sheet on top of that, then another waterproof protector on top of that before a final, second sheet on top. This means that all you need to do is whip off the top wet sheet and protector and the bed is clean and dry again, with no need to hunt out and fit clean sheets in the middle of the night. Other standard advice is to limit the amount your child has to drink in the evening and to make sure that they go to the toilet before bed. Some people find some success with waking their children just enough to take them to the toilet when they go to bed. My biggest tip is not to rush night-time dryness; it's much easier to put a child in nappies at night than it is to have to get up and change sheets and pyjamas.

As mentioned previously, bed-wetting is totally normal for children under the age of seven, and it is absolutely not a problem if your child still needs to wear nappies at night at this age.

Chapter 2

Sleep throughout history and the impact of modern life

've often wondered if parents in other cultures – and at different points in history – struggle as much with their children's sleep as we do. Is night waking, early rising and refusing to nap common in other cultures, and more prevalent now than it was in the past? Or have they always been universal problems? I've always found learning how parents from other countries take care of their families fascinating and, increasingly, I have become interested in the history of parenting. We can learn a lot from both.

Sleep throughout history

Segmented sleep

One element of historical sleep behaviour that I find fascinating is the practice of segmented sleep. One of the foremost experts on this is Professor Roger Ekirch, a historian at Virginia University in the US. Over the last twenty years, Professor Ekirch has studied the historical practice of sleeping in two distinct segments, with a period of time awake in between. His research tells us that it is only in the last couple of hundred years or so that people have 'slept through the night' in one single block. Indeed, the practice of first and second sleeps can be traced back to ancient Greek civilisations, with many further references occurring throughout history. Professor Ekirch suggests that it is only since the dawn of industrialised civilisations, and the introduction of artificial light, that our sleep has been focused on one long, uninterrupted block.

Professor Ekirch's research into segmented sleep has found that for most the 'first sleep' began roughly two hours after sunset. This period of sleep would last around four hours, followed by around two hours of being awake and active. This was followed by the 'second sleep', with waking occurring with the rising of the sun. Professor Ekirch's research has unearthed over five hundred mentions of segmented sleep throughout history, but as he says, 'It's not just the number of references – it is the way they refer to it, as if it was common knowledge.' He suggests that many of today's 'sleep problems' are not problems at all, but a response to the relatively modern practice of taking one single block of sleep per night. In an online article in *BBC News* magazine in 2012, psychologist Gregg Jacobs commented on Professor Ekirch's research saying, 'For most of evolution we slept a certain way; waking up during the night is part of normal human physiology. The idea that we must sleep in a consolidated block could be damaging if it makes people who wake up at night anxious, as this anxiety can itself prohibit sleep and is likely to seep into waking life, too.' In the same piece, Professor Russell Foster, a neuroscientist at Oxford University, states, 'Many people wake up at night and panic. I tell them that what they are experiencing is a throwback to the bi-modal sleep pattern.'

Nobody knows why people chose to sleep in two distinct chunks in the past. There are some suggestions that the waking period between the two sleeps was used for prayer and creative thought, and sex was common in these periods of awakening. Whatever the reason, it appears that for most of our history sleeping in two separate phases was normal and it is our new practice of taking one long sleep at night that is abnormal.

With this in mind I can't help but think about the times my own children woke in the night, usually between 1 and 3am (the time that would usually have been the period between first and second sleeps), seemingly wide awake and not in the least bit interested in going back to sleep. For most of the last two thousand years it seems this nocturnal behaviour would have been completely normal. This doesn't necessarily make it any easier to cope when you are exhausted and desperate for your children to calm down, but it may help to make some sense of their behaviour.

Modern inhibitors of sleep

There have been a number of other changes in our lives in the past few centuries that could be having an impact on our sleep and that of our children. There are four main culprits: the use of artificial lighting, our ever-growing use of screens, daycare and pre-school and the process of putting our clocks forward and back. Let's look at these in a little more detail.

Artificial light

Electric lighting is such a commonplace part of our lives today that it is hard to imagine what life was like without it. In my opinion, no modern invention has changed the way we sleep today as much as the light bulb. For thousands of years our circadian rhythms were governed by the rising and setting of the sun, with melatonin release increasing from dusk and cortisol increasing with the breaking of dawn. This is how we are supposed to function. The delicate and finely tuned process of our body's response to light is amazing; is it any wonder then that things go awry after we introduce artificial light sources? Now it can be as light as day for twenty-four hours a day. Even if we sleep without a light on we still have artificially lit evenings and many children sleep with the glow of a night light. Scientists call external time cues, such as the use of electric light, *zeitgebers* (German for 'time givers'), because of their effects on our body clocks.

According to Charles Czeisler, Professor of Sleep Medicine at Harvard Medical School, 'There are many reasons why people get insufficient sleep in our 24/7 society. But the precipitating factor is an often unappreciated, technological breakthrough: the electric light ... light affects our circadian rhythms more powerfully than any drug.' In his research, Professor Czeisler found that between the years 1950 and 2000 the use of artificial light increased fourfold and, as you might imagine, sleeping problems have increased correspondingly. On average, children are now getting 1.2 hours less sleep at night than they did one hundred years ago. He comments, 'Technology has effectively decoupled us from the natural 24-hour day to which our bodies evolved, driving us to go to bed later. And we use caffeine in the morning to rise as early as we ever did, putting the squeeze on sleep.'[1]

Interestingly, a study at the University of Colorado into the effects of camping in nature found that even one week without the interruption of electric lighting can be enough to improve sleep. The researchers found that seven days of camping, with exposure only to the natural light of the sun and moon, and camp-fires in the evening, is enough to reset our circadian rhythms to be more in-line with the natural sunrise and sunset.

After studying the melatonin levels of the participants, the researchers found that levels began to rise around two hours earlier when camping, compared to when they were at home surrounded by artificial light.[2] We are keen campers in our family and I always feel rested after a week sleeping under canvas, despite the discomfort.

Red light, blue light

You could argue that we have used artificial lighting for hundreds of years, in the form of candles and fire, but there is one important difference – the colour and intensity of the light. Modern lighting is incredibly bright and, importantly, focused on the blue and white colour spectrum. The colour of natural sources of light, such as fire and candlelight, is always orange–red. Why is this important? Research into the impact of different colours of light has found our body's natural clock system responds differently to artificial light sources, depending on the colour.[3] Speaking about her research into the effect of colour wavelengths of light and their impact on melatonin, Debra Skene, a scientist from the University of Surrey, says, 'We observed peak light sensitivity at a wavelength of around 460 to 480 nanometres – a nice deep blue.' She goes on, 'Red light, by contrast, has only a weak impact on melanopsin receptors and is less prone to stimulate wakefulness. So adjusting the relative levels of blue and red light that people are exposed to throughout the day could preserve normal circadian timing even during prolonged exposure to artificial light.'[4]

The impact of red and blue light on circadian rhythms is being tested by a team of researchers from Boston and Pennsylvania, using astronauts based at the International Space Station. The light and dark cycle experienced by astronauts in orbit lasts for only around ninety minutes, which is too short for the circadian rhythms to function correctly. Understandably, this causes all sorts of problems for the astronauts. The research aims to test the effects of using artificial blue and red light sources over a twenty-four-hour period, in order to attempt to simulate a circadian rhythm similar to what the astronauts would experience on Earth. This research is in its early stages, but it may have huge implications for how we light our homes, reducing the negative impact of artificial light on our sleep/wake cycles.

I wonder what effect using dim, red-based lighting sources in the evening and bright, blue-based lighting in the daytime would have upon the sleep of babies and young children. Currently most children's night lights employ a white- or blue-based light source. If the night light has different colour settings, parents often select the blue one, as they feel that this colour is soothing and may aid their child's sleep. Biologically, it could be doing quite the opposite. It is also interesting to note the difference in colour spectrum of the older-style incandescent bulbs in comparison to the new, blue-based, energy-saving light bulbs. Could these modern light bulbs potentially cause more sleep problems than their less efficient predecessors? Professor Richard Stevens, an epidemiologist from the University of Connecticut, believes this is the case and said, in a *Daily Mail* article in October 2013, 'In the evening, an incandescent bulb is better than an energy-saving fluorescent bulb. There's been a recent push to phase out incandescent bulbs in favour of energy-saving bulbs, but although they may be more energy efficient, they produce a lot of blue light.'

With this in mind, the obvious answer is to get as much natural light in the daytime as possible, using blue-based artificial light sources where necessary. In the morning, open the curtains as early as you can and get outside every single day for at least fifteen minutes when the day is at its brightest. In the evening, observe the natural light changes and when dusk begins to fall, dim the lights and change to more red-based light sources, particularly in the nursery. If possible, remove light sources altogether from the room your baby or child sleeps in, but if they do need a night light, try to find one on the red colour spectrum. A good alternative to buying a child's night light is to use an ordinary lamp fitted with a low-watt, red incandescent (not energy saving) light bulb in it.

As well as considering your nursery lighting, think about the lighting used in your bathroom. Most babies and young children spend several minutes in a very brightly lit bathroom immediately before bedtime every night, often taking a 'relaxing' bath – ironically in a light that is known to stimulate their bodies. With this in mind, I use orange- and pink-coloured, battery-powered, rechargeable candles in my bathroom in the evening. Taking a bath with them dotted around the room is a very relaxing experience, not just for my children but for me too.

Screen time

Another facet of modern life that is playing havoc with our sleep and that of our children is electronic screen time. We spend hours each week looking at the television, tablets, computers and smart phones. There seems to be a trend at the moment for designing tablets and other electronic devices for children and even babies, not to mention the vast array of apps designed to entertain children. Moreover, the advent of satellite, cable and free-to-view TV means that children's television programmes are broadcast almost twenty-four hours per day, in contrast to the two hours per day shown when we were children. There is no denying the fact that our children spend many more hours per day in front of an electronic screen than any other generation and this is only likely to grow. What effect, if any, does this have upon our children's sleep? The answer is 'a lot' and it isn't just sleep that suffers.

Research conducted in New Zealand in 2013 found that in the last hour and a half before bedtime almost 50 per cent of children watch as much as half an hour of television. Unsurprisingly, those children who watched television in the last hour or two before bedtime went to sleep later than those who watched none.[5] Similar effects have been found when children play computer games in the run-up to bedtime. Louise Foley, lead researcher, commented that 'Reducing screen time in this pre-sleep window could be a good strategy for helping kids go to sleep earlier.' Speaking about this research, Professor Christakis, a paediatrician at the University of Washington, said, 'There is growing evidence that media use around sleep time is bad for sleep initiation: it's not so much having a bedtime for your children. You have to have a bedtime for their devices.' In my house all 'screen time' ends at 7pm and my children have to check-in their electronic devices with me for the night. We also have a total ban on any electronic screens in bedrooms.

Regarding television viewing, many parents comment that they find it good for their child to 'wind down' and say that they only allow their children to watch special bedtime-related programmes. I know when you have more than one child that television makes your evenings easier, as the 'electronic babysitter' entertains them while you cook dinner or bathe the baby, but it's important to be aware that television can have a negative effect, irrespective of how age-appropriate the programme is. Programmes aimed at children are still screen time and that in itself makes the child's mind too active, while the harsh blue screen lighting inhibits their circadian rhythms.

Other forms of screen time, including computers, tablets and laptops, can have an equally damaging effect on sleep. The effects are similar to that of television viewing; namely that the light emitted from the devices promotes brain activity. Research carried out in 2013 found that the more children used electronic media the less sleep they got. The lead researcher, Teija

Nuutinen, commented that 'Media viewing habits should be considered for kids who are tired and struggling to concentrate, or who have behaviour problems caused by lack of sleep.'[6]

The most sensible advice is therefore to keep the last two hours before bedtime completely screen-free, so no smart phones, tablets and computers, but also no television viewing, irrespective of the programme. If you have trouble sleeping, this advice applies to you just as much as your child.

Daycare and pre-school

Electronic screens and artificial light aside, there is one very important difference in our modern lifestyles that has a profound impact on a child's sleep: daycare. Being looked after outside the home is a very recent development in our society and one that is increasingly common, as parents both return to work, single parent families increase and we parent away from our extended families. With many more free pre-school places becoming available for younger children, more and more children under the age of five are spending a significant part of their day away from home. Ninety-six per cent of parents of three- and four-year-olds take advantage of funded pre-school places; figures that have steadily risen in the last ten years. Two-thirds of these children attend pre-school for the maximum of thirteen hours per week.

The impact of daycare on naps

Current figures suggest that around 21 per cent of children under two years of age attend a daycare setting (many more are cared for by nannies, childminders and grandparents). This is a figure that the government appears keen to increase. This brightly lit, busy, stimulating environment is not one that babies and toddlers have been exposed to before, historically speaking, and research now is taking place to ascertain the effects. Rather than delve into the pros and cons of different forms of childcare, in the context of sleep, I'm interested in looking at how the sleep of these 20 per cent of under two-year-olds and over 90 per cent of three- and four-year-olds may be affected by this extended period spent outside of their home being care for by others. There are two main potential effects worth considering when looking at the impact of daycare on the under-fives: the effect on the natural nap times of children and the impact of cortisol on the child's circadian rhythms.

Research published in 2013, looking at the impact of daycare on naps of pre-school-aged children, found that the lack of naps taken by children once they started pre-school could be negatively affecting not just their sleep, but also their learning.[7] These results were obviously more important for those children who still naturally napped during the day, which for three- and four-year-olds is estimated to be somewhere between 25 and 50 per cent. The lead researcher, Laura Kurdziel, commented, 'when they miss a nap, the child cannot recover this benefit of sleep with their overnight sleep. It seems that there is an additional benefit of having the sleep occur in close proximity to the learning. Children should not only be given the opportunity, they should be encouraged to sleep by creating an environment which supports sleep.'

The impact of daycare on circadian rhythms

Perhaps more important is the impact of daycare and pre-school on a child's cortisol levels and circadian rhythms. An analysis of nine different studies, looking at the effects of daycare upon cortisol levels of young children, found that children in daycare have higher cortisol levels than children looked after in a home setting. Not only was the level higher for children in daycare, their levels also rose over the course of the day and were higher in the afternoon, an effect that was not seen in those children at home. This effect was the most noticeable for under-three-year-olds.

The researchers commented, 'We speculate that children in daycare show elevated cortisol levels because of their stressful interactions in a group setting.'[8] I'm not sure this is the whole story. I wonder if their cortisol levels were elevated more because of a combination of disrupted nap times and brightly lit rooms. This would disrupt their circadian rhythms and only add to the stress of the constant stimulation of their surroundings and exposure to a number of different adults and children.

Whatever the cause of the raised cortisol levels, this research is useful for parents who work and use daycare. Knowing that your child's hormone levels will stimulate them to be awake and active when you collect them at the end of the day should help you to tailor the evening routine. It is commonly thought that young children need at least two to three hours at home in a calming environment for their cortisol levels to fall sufficiently for their bodies to realise it is time for sleep. It is vital that these hours at home in the evening are as non-stimulating as possible, with light and electronic screens kept to a minimum and any play kept calm. Often parents finish a busy and stressful day at work, collect their child at around 6pm on the way home and are eager to get their child to bed so they can relax. This can often mean that children are put to bed long before their cortisol levels reach a low enough level to sleep. It's no wonder that bedtimes can be protracted and exhausting for all involved. For a child in daycare, delaying bedtime until two to three hours after they arrive home can often result in a longer and calmer night's sleep and easier bedtime. Ultimately this gives the parent more 'me-time', just perhaps not at the time they might want it. There is no magic answer here; it comes back to balancing the pressures of modern-day life with those of an infant who has primal needs and biology.

Daylight saving and foreign travel

Two more facets of modern life, namely daylight saving and long-haul travel, also have negative effects on normal baby and child sleep.

Daylight saving was first proposed at the end of the nineteenth century in order to give us lighter afternoons and evenings. The aim was to enable farmers to work later in the day; promote more outdoor leisure time; save coal during the First World War; and reduce the usage of incandescent light bulbs, and thus electricity. The practice was established in the UK in 1916, with clocks being put forward one hour on the last Sunday of March and put back on the last Sunday in October.

Although daylight-saving changes are usually fairly well tolerated by most adults, things are less positive for parents of small children. Research published in 2008 indicated that the daylight-saving time 'enhanced night-time restlessness' and 'compromised the quality of sleep.'[9] Although this research was conducted on adults, it indicates how daylight saving affects human biology. Sadly, to date, no research of this kind has been conducted on children.

How to help your child cope with clock changes

Babies and young toddlers understandably have no concept of daylight saving or the fact they are now expected to go to sleep one hour early or wake one hour later. The only way that you can help your child to adjust to the new time setting is to introduce it very gradually. Starting two weeks before the clocks change, move your child's bedtime forward or backwards (depending on which way the clocks are changing) by five minutes each day, with the aim of building up to the full hour's difference by the end of the fortnight. This can work fairly well, but often it doesn't make any difference to the child's wake time in the morning.

Jet lag and crossing time zones

The last of the modern practices that cause sleep problems is that of long-haul travel. The invention of commercial aeroplanes has created so many opportunities for long-distance travel in the last eighty years, but we pay a price for this in the form of jet lag. International travel plays havoc with our circadian rhythms, but as adults we can rationalise what is happening and try to stay awake or sleep earlier in order to try to compensate. Babies and young children simply do not have the ability to do this, making it harder to cope with them during long-haul travel.

Jet lag: top tips for under-fives

- If possible, try to avoid travelling to countries with large time differences, sticking to those with up to a three-hour difference when your children are young.

- Consider delaying the trip if possible until your child is old enough to understand the concept of different time zones and you can encourage them to adjust their behaviour to the new time.

- Keep at least three days either side of the journey as clear as possible; this means not planning very much for the first three days of your holiday, or when returning home.

- Consider trying to shift your child's sleep times in advance of the trip, in a similar way to the method I have suggested for daylight saving changes (see page 44).

- Consider flying overnight, in the hope that your child will sleep, making the flight as easy as possible, and arriving in daylight, making the following day easier.

- Keep the nights as dark as possible and get outside as soon as you can in the mornings, to allow your child's circadian rhythms the best chance to adjust to the new time zone.

- Be understanding of what your child is going through and realise that during this unsettling period they are likely to need your comfort more than usual, both in the night and in the day.

Ending this chapter by looking at international travel is fitting, as the next chapter examines how infant and child sleep is handled by different cultures.

Chapter 3

Sleep around the world – and how other parents cope

I am fascinated by anthropology, or the study of humankind, particularly the parenting practices of other cultures. I often wonder what we can learn from them and incorporate into Western life to make parenting easier for us. When it comes to sleep, I think we can learn a lot.

There are four parenting practices from other cultures that I believe could help our children sleep better. These are:

- the practice of siestas and later bedtimes

- the carrying of babies and young toddlers and allowing them to nap while in physical contact with us

- sharing a bed or room with our children

- a respect for motherhood and the support given to parents of young children.

Let's look at each of these in turn.

Siestas and later bedtimes

Have you ever been on holiday to a warm country and decided to go shopping after lunch, only to be faced with row upon row of closed shops? The practice of taking an afternoon siesta is common in countries with a high average temperature, where the afternoon heat makes it difficult to do much else. Research in 2006 suggested that the practice of taking an afternoon siesta might be due, in part, to the glucose contained in our lunch, which inhibits neurons in the brain that are responsible for keeping us alert and active. The researchers said: 'It has been known for a while that people and animals can become sleepy and less active after a meal, but brain signals responsible for this were poorly understood. We have pinpointed how glucose – the sugar in food – can stop brain cells from producing signals that keep us awake ... This may well provide an explanation for after-meal tiredness and why it is difficult to sleep when hungry ... This research perhaps sheds light on why our European friends are so fond of their siestas.'[1]

When it comes to feelings of alertness, scientists at the Loughborough University Sleep Research Centre have found that taking an afternoon nap is more effective than drinking caffeine or sleeping-in for an extra hour and a half in the morning. Further benefits may include protection against heart disease, as indicated by a study from Athens University in 2007. Speaking about this research, Dr Michael Twery, Director of the National Heart Lung and Blood Institute's National Centre on Sleep Disorders Research, said: 'Napping may help deal with the stress of daily living. Another possibility is that it is part of the normal biological rhythm of daily living. The biological clock that drives sleep and wakefulness has two cycles each day, and one of them dips usually in the early afternoon. It's possible that not engaging in napping for some people might disrupt these processes.'[2]

Could it be that siestas are not only beneficial for us, but a normal part of our biology? Afternoon naps may not just be important for children, making sure that their sleep needs are met, but they could be important for adults too, particularly as a way of consolidating our own sleep when we have a baby or toddler waking at night.

The practice of taking a siesta often goes hand in hand with a much later bedtime for children. Again, this is common in countries with a warmer climate. Research conducted in 2013 found that pre-school-aged children from Asian countries tend to have a much later bedtime than those from Europe, the USA and Australasia. The earliest bedtimes were found in Australia and New Zealand, with an average bedtime of 7.43pm. In stark contrast, bedtimes in India averaged 10.26pm, almost three hours later! Daytime naps, however, were more common in the Asian countries studied, but the total time asleep per twenty-four hours was roughly the same for all children, no matter where they lived. It appears that the children from Asian countries were spreading their sleeps throughout the day and night, whereas in the predominantly Caucasian countries daytime naps were significantly rarer and more sleep was being taken at night.[3]

Later bedtimes are prevalent in many other cultures around the world, particularly amongst African tribes. Anthropologists Carol Worthman and Melissa Melby described the different bedtime habits of two such tribes, the !Kung and the Efe, in a 2002 article, saying: 'neither Kung nor Efe have bedtimes, so time of falling asleep varies widely with individuals. People stay up as long as something interesting – a conversation, music, dance – is happening and participate; then they go to sleep when they feel like it ... Additionally no one, including children, is told to go to bed, and individuals of any age may nod off amid ongoing social intercourse and fade in and out of sleep during night-time social activities.'[4] This social night-time behaviour is not just limited to African tribes. In many parts of South America, and in Indonesia, children are included in social interactions just as much as adults and often have no set bedtime or have one that is significantly later than much of Europe, North America, Canada and Australasia. Worthman and Melby also looked at the practices of families in Bali, Indonesia, observing: 'Balinese, who engage in extensive night-time ritual activity, bring children along with them to all rituals, where they may fall asleep at will, although in this case they must learn to stay awake as adults. In other words, bedtimes are not fixed and sleep–wake boundaries are rather fluid.'

These later, more fluid, bedtimes may be more in line with the normal biological needs of children than the earlier rigid bedtimes enforced by many societies. Research in 2013 studied toddler bedtimes in comparison to melatonin levels and found that, for many toddlers, their sleep problems could be caused by parents putting them to bed too early. They found that some toddlers had later melatonin rises than others and if those toddlers were put to bed before their melatonin levels had risen appropriately then sleep problems were likely. Conversely, the study found that toddlers who experienced a longer interval between the onset of their melatonin release and their bedtime fell asleep more quickly and protested at bedtime far less. The research found that the average timing of melatonin rises in toddlers occurred at around 7.40pm. Researcher Monique LeBourgeois commented on the results of the study: 'Sleeping at the wrong "biological clock" time leads to sleep difficulties, like insomnia, in adults. This study is the first to show that a poor fit between bedtimes selected by the parents of toddlers and the rise in their evening melatonin production increases their likelihood of night-time settling difficulties.' She added, 'We believe that arming parents with knowledge about the biological clock can help them make optimal choices about their child's activities before bedtime, at bedtime, and his or her sleeping environment.'[5]

I wonder if, in part, some of our difficulties with our children's sleeping behaviour arise because we expect them to go to bed earlier than they are ready to. I know evenings are precious, particularly when you have been at work all day, but I can't help thinking that we may be creating more problems for ourselves by trying to get our children to sleep too early.

Carrying infants throughout the day

Have you ever seen a photograph of an African mother carrying her baby on her back in a brightly coloured piece of fabric? Or perhaps a Mexican mother carrying a sleeping toddler in a woven rebozo? For many cultures, carrying young children is a way of life and most daytime naps are taken in whatever is used to carry the child. Barbara Wishingrad describes her observations of mothers in Mexico in her article on 'In arms parenting': 'Every time I got on a bus to go anywhere, women with babies tied on surrounded me. They wore them in a wrap called a rebozo. They climbed on, sat down or remained standing, stuffed bags into overhead racks, talked to their neighbours or older children and climbed off. The babies nursed, slept, looked around, and moved with their mothers.' This idea is echoed in the book *Bless the Baby* by Melanie Waxman: 'In many cultures, women have carried babies on their backs ... Babies are comforted by being close to their mother and are rocked as she moves. The confined space in the carrier creates a feeling of safety.'

In *Childhood: A Multicultural View* (see Bibliography), Melvin Konner describes the normality of almost constant physical contact between mother and child and speculates about how it protected the child in times past. 'In hunting and gathering societies like the Baka and the !Kung, infants are carried by the mother most of the time, and are nursed several times an hour ... these seemingly strange things are also true of our closest monkey and ape relatives ... During our evolution, the constant closeness served several functions; mothers stood between babies and creatures that might eat them; they kept the babies warm with the warmth of their own bodies.' In *A World of Babies: Imagined Childcare Guides for Seven Societies*, anthropologist Dr Alma Gottlieb discusses how the Beng in the Ivory Coast, in the south-west of Africa, handle their infants' naps. 'Among the Beng, village farmers living in the Cote d'Ivoire, babies spend their days on someone's back; either the mother or a designated baby carrier. Carrying a baby in this way is considered a good way to get babies to fall asleep.'

Research by Urs Hunziker and Ronald Barr found that babies who were carried during the daytime for one hour more than those in the control group cried 43 per cent less. Between the hours of 4pm to midnight the babies who were carried more cried 51 per cent less, compared to a control group.[6] From a baby's point of view, being carried makes them feel safe and secure; being close to the wearer's heart provides a reassuring noise, similar to that heard in utero; the scent is familiar and reassuring and they are kept warm. Add to this the constant, subtle movements caused by the wearer's breathing and the large, rocking and bouncing-type movements when the wearer is walking and it's no wonder that they are significantly calmer. For all of these reasons, using a good baby sling or carrier, with the baby facing inwards only, to reduce stimulation and hold the back and hips in a physiologically correct and comfortable position, can provide much needed nap-time relief for both baby and parent.

Another added benefit of carrying your baby during naps is that you can still play with their older brother or sister, if they have one, and you can get on with things if you want to. Carrying during daytime naps isn't just for small babies: if you buy a good, supportive carrier (from a specialist retailer) you can carry your child right into the toddler years and beyond; older children usually being carried on the wearer's back, like the African babies mentioned at the start of this section. The benefits don't end there though. Scientists from the Infant Sleep Information Source (ISIS, see Bibliography) suggest that taking naps in slings can help to keep babies safe and at less risk of SIDS: 'The advice for new parents is that your baby should sleep in the same room as you, day and night, until they are at least six months old. Studies have shown this to reduce the risk of SIDS. An English study, comparing 325 SIDS babies with 1300 control babies, found that 75 per cent of the day-time SIDS deaths occurred while babies were alone in a room. Using a sling or baby carrier may make it easier for you to keep your baby close during the day.'

If you share the common concern of many parents, that this may create bad habits that will be difficult to break at a later stage, one conclusion of the team at ISIS may offer some reassurance: 'Studies show that babies need to have positive sleep associations and that babies whose sleep environment is calm, and for whom going to sleep is pleasant, will develop better long-term sleeping habits. For some babies a calm and pleasant sleep environment involves being in contact with their mother or other caregiver – a typical practice in many countries. Some babies therefore prefer to settle by being soothed by their parents, and not by being left alone, so these babies fall asleep happily in a sling.' So if your child is small enough for you to carry them easily in a sling for their naps, they sleep well and you are happy with the arrangement, then keep doing it. We waste so much time worrying about the future that we cause ourselves all sort of heartache in the present. The irony is that half the things we worry about that 'might happen' never do and, while hindsight is wonderful, it would be much better to use a tool to help you with your child's sleep now, than reminisce a few months or years down the line that it would have worked quite well.

Bedsharing and co-sleeping

'The more touch a child gets in childhood, the calmer he is likely to be as an adult.' These wise words are from Professor Margot Sunderland, director of the Centre for Child Mental Health in the UK. Like many psychologists, Professor Sunderland supports both bedsharing and co-sleeping (the former being sharing a bed with your child and the latter being sharing a room with your child, although confusingly bedsharing is also commonly referred to as co-sleeping by many). In her book *What Every Parent Needs to Know*, she says, 'Extensive scientific research shows that safe co-sleeping can be a real investment for your child's future physical and emotional health.' Commenting on the safety of sharing a bed with your child, she says: 'In China, where co-sleeping is taken for granted, SIDS is so rare it doesn't even have a name ... SIDS is also uncommon among the populations of South East Asia, such as those of Vietnam, Cambodia and Thailand, where nearly all babies sleep with their parents. In Hong Kong, where high-density living makes co-sleeping the norm, rates of SIDS are among the lowest in the world.' The science and practicalities of co-sleeping and bedsharing are examined in Chapter 6, but for now I would like to concentrate on the cultural aspects of sharing a bed or a room with your child.

In 1992, researchers studied the different sleeping patterns of middle-class Caucasian, American mothers and Guatemalan, Mayan mothers.[7] Their findings revealed that all of the Mayan mothers in their research shared a bed with their babies, while the Mayan fathers shared a bed with their toddlers. The American sample was unsurprisingly very different, with none of the sample sleeping with their children; however most were sharing a bedroom with their baby in its own crib, until the age of six months, in order to 'make sure that they were still breathing'. After six months, however, the American mothers felt that the babies needed to learn to be independent and moved them to their own bedrooms. The Mayan mothers, on the other hand, felt that sleeping in close proximity to their children was the 'reasonable way' for the family to sleep. Researchers found that Mayan babies may breastfeed during the night until they are two to three years old.

Dr T. Berry Brazelton found similar results in 1990. Commenting on Japanese culture and the frequency of bedsharing in Japan he said, 'the Japanese think the US culture rather merciless in pushing small children toward such independence at night'.[8] These culturally based trends have continued to echo through scientific and anthropological research for the last twenty years. Another study of Japanese culture in 2005, noted the tendency to both bedshare and co-sleep: 'In Japan, family members have traditionally slept in the same room, and many babies sleep in with their parents. The traditional Japanese arrangement of co-sleeping represents an environment in which parents are readily accessible to children during waking episodes.'[9]

Interestingly, research conducted in 2011, which looked at the sleep of Japanese children from birth to three years of age in comparison with the sleep of children of the same age from other Asian countries, found that 'Young children in Japan exhibited significantly fewer nocturnal wakings' and that 'sleep problems were reported by significantly fewer parents in Japan compared with those in other Asian countries/regions.'[10] The research in this case focused only on night wakings and durations of sleep, but I wonder if the cultural trend of bedsharing and co-sleeping was significantly higher amongst the Japanese children than those from the other countries studied. Similar findings were produced by a 2013 study comparing the sleep of Asian and Caucasian families. The researchers reported that 'Mothers in predominantly Asian countries/regions had ... decreased number and duration of night wakings, more night-time sleep, and more total sleep than mothers from predominantly Caucasian countries.'[11] Again, I can't help but speculate about the effects of bedsharing and co-sleeping, knowing how it is considered normal and is widely practised throughout Asia. As research conducted in 2010 found, 'For predominantly Caucasian, the most common behaviour occurring at bedtime is falling asleep independently in own crib/bed (57%), compared to just 4% of those children living in predominantly Asian regions.'[12] Is the practice of bedsharing and co-sleeping the biggest variable in terms of the Asian families sleeping better at night?

In his book *Childhood: A Multicultural View*, Melvin Konner comments, 'From Africa to the Arctic to the Americas, modern-day hunter-gatherers keep their babies in close, physical contact throughout the day, and mothers typically sleep with them at night. Babies frequently fall asleep while breastfeeding and experiencing skin-to-skin contact.' In her article 'Never Leave your Little One Alone: Raising an Ifaluk child', Professor of Psychology Huynh-Nhu Le looks at the sleeping practices of the inhabitants of the Ifaluk islands in Micronesia (from *A World of Babies*). She comments: 'Among the Ifaluk of the South Pacific, babies sleep alongside their parents each night. This continues until they are about three years old. During the day, babies may be rocked to sleep.'

The practice of sharing a family bed or a room is seen all around the world. Research published in 2013 focused on family sleeping patterns in Egypt, concentrating on children aged three and older. The researchers concluded that 'co-sleeping was prevalent' and provided 'more regular, and less disrupted sleep'.[13] These findings echoed earlier research into Egyptian sleeping patterns, which found that 'Of recorded sleep events, 69% involved co-sleeping, 24% included more than one co-sleeper, and only 21% were solitary.' Once again the researchers found that 'Co-sleepers had fewer night arousals.'[14]

Given the prevalence in other countries of sharing a bed or

room with children, you have to wonder why it is so frowned upon in many parts of Western society, particularly when it helps everyone to get more sleep. It may be that our preference for sleeping apart from our children when they are still very young is a major cause of many sleep problems.

Supporting young families

Perhaps the most important difference between parenting in our society and in other cultures is our view of young families, mothers in particular, and the lack of support provided for them. Only a century ago it was the norm to be a stay-at-home mother; it was rightly seen as an important job. This is no longer the case – a fact that is all too evident in the actions of politicians, who are keen to get as many mothers back into the workforce and children into daycare as quickly as possible, in order to increase domestic productivity and bolster the economy. This is exacerbated by the immense pressure on the modern, nuclear family to 'have it all' – a pressure largely contributable to the media, who expect new mothers to lose their baby weight and become a 'yummy mummy', with a perfect figure, a perfect house, perfect clothes and a perfect job. It is, however, not possible to live up to this ideal while responding to the normal and natural needs of our infants. Add to this the fact that we now parent miles away from our extended families, with no support network, and it's clear that something has to give. Sadly, very often, it is the needs of our children, or our own sanity. We sleep-train our children in order that they fit into our modern lives more easily; we fool ourselves into believing that it is our offspring that have 'sleep problems', rather than opening our eyes to the real problem – the disharmony between the primal needs of our young and the expectations of the modern world. Who really has the problem?

Sometimes it is the mental and physical health of the parents that suffers when they try to balance the constant needs of their children with the demands of modern life. Many mothers in particular feel guilty for having negative thoughts about their children, especially at times when they are not sleeping. This is summed up so well by this mother in psychotherapist Dana Breen's book *Talking with Mothers*: 'It was a pinnacle of depression that I reached. I have a feeling that was what started it. Leo would just not go to bed at night any more and I've been used to having no problems putting him to bed at seven o'clock and then for over a week it was half past ten, eleven o'clock, half past eleven and up at five, and there was no way I could carry on; and I thought "Oh my God", I thought things got better as they went on – but he went backwards. I'm saying "I don't even have my evenings now, I've got nothing left".' Like many mothers today, this mother desperately needed more support, from her family, friends or paid-for. For most, this help is either not available (in the case of family and friends) or simply just not affordable (in the case of paid-for help).

Even when help is available, parents often feel either too embarrassed or too guilty to ask for it, feeling that it may demonstrate their inability to be a good mother or father. Remember that your child's sleep has nothing to do with your parenting abilities and you should *never* be afraid to ask for help. We are simply not meant to parent in the way we do today – alone, unsupported and juggling different roles and the demands of modern life. I love Professor Margot Sunderland's take on this, when she says, 'Babies are awful sleepers. When we accept this, maybe we will stop seeing a wakeful baby as some kind of parental failure.' I agree wholeheartedly with her sentiment, but I would include young children as well as babies.

Returning to Leo's mother, she found a way to cope with her child's wakefulness. As in most cases the answer didn't lie in changing her child, it lay in changing her lifestyle and support network, by returning to work part-time and hiring a nanny. In short, she was better able to cope with her son's needs by first taking care of her own. After her return to work and with the nanny firmly settled in, she says: 'I appreciate him so much more ... I'm much more relaxed, much happier. Life's more hectic but I prefer it that way ... I can't really lose my temper with him, which I was quite capable of doing before. I find it difficult to get cross with him, I tend to laugh at situations now whereas before it took very little and I'd get it all out of proportion. I'm just not made to stay at home all day, I've decided.' I think in many cases this is true, but with the addition of the word 'alone' – 'I'm just not made to stay at home all day *alone*'. We are not meant to shoulder all of the responsibility of parenting alone so, when we do, it is almost impossible to cope unless we are blessed with an abnormally 'good' sleeper.

In her book *Mother and Child*, Deborah Jackson comments on the concept of the popular phrase, 'It takes a village to raise a child', saying 'Throughout history, human beings have been interdependent, forming intimate networks of trust; asking for assistance when they need it and knowing that help, without judgement is on hand ... Generations of multi-tasking mothers have managed to combine childcare and other work without gadgets, supermarkets and automobiles. Instead, they rely on each other. Babies are raised not by one mother alone, but by a team of mothers and helpers.' This lack of a supportive 'village' in our society often adds to feelings of helplessness about our situation, with parents wondering what they did wrong to create a child with such poor sleeping habits. In reality, though, it is often shortcomings in our own lives and greater society that are more to blame.

In her book *What Mothers Do*, fittingly in a chapter entitled 'So tired I could die', psychotherapist Naomi Stadlen says, 'Modern society is not organised to facilitate the transition women have to make when they become mothers. It's a momentous change. New mothers often cope by telling themselves to expect motherhood to be challenging at first, but then it will get easier. It certainly does get easier. But not automatically. It becomes easier when mothers take leave of their old lives, and adjust to the new.' Stadlen contrasts the role of motherhood in Western society to that of societies where mothers are more supported and respected, saying 'In traditional societies, mothers' responsibilities are usually shared, and a mother's female relatives are expected to help her. But in modern societies these relatives are usually not available. They are more likely to be in full-time employment ... Mothers who still live with traditional families report that the responsibilities are spread among their female relatives. Someone takes the baby while they sleep and they get plenty of practical help.'

Speaking of the support received in other cultures, Deborah Jackson writes in her book *Three in a Bed*, 'In her family village, the Pakistani woman can count on the support of her in-laws and cousins when bringing up her children. Following the birth of a baby, she is exempted from all household duties – other than feeding and caring for her child – for forty days ... In urban society, where many people live alone, drive to work alone and eat alone, people have to fend for themselves.' Professor Huynh-Nhu Le echoes the same sentiments when discussing the value of children and parenthood amongst the Ifaluk islanders of the South Pacific, who take a similarly supportive view to family life. 'Children are precious to the Ifaluk people, and everyone shares the responsibility for their upbringing – socialisation is not the exclusive domain of a child's parents.'

There is no doubt that we are parenting dramatically differently today than we were just half a century ago, and in a way that is at odds with practices in other cultures. This style of isolated, unsupported parenting is taking its toll on us. Quite simply, we're not meant to do it this way. We invent all manner of techniques, products and medications to help get our children to sleep, in order that our modern lives are less tiring and less stressful, when in fact the real key lies in challenging the way we live our lives.

The truth is our children probably sleep no differently to those in traditional Asian or African villages, or those who lived in our own country two hundred years ago, but for those parents the vital difference lies in the support network around them. The real problem is the disharmony between the primal needs of our young and the expectations and demands of parenting in the modern world, hand in hand with our relatively recent manipulation of light and dark and the ever increasing use of technology. Perhaps the real question to ask is not 'How do we fix our child's sleep problem?' but 'How can we help our children to fit into a modern world which is not in harmony with their biology or psychological needs?' In Chapter 6 I examine ways that we as parents can ease the burden somewhat and nurture ourselves more so that these new, unrealistic demands are a little easier to cope with.

I'd like to end this chapter with a story from a mother who has really taken on board the anthropological aspects of sleep and used what she has learnt from other cultures to help her own family. (Despite sharing a name, this is not my own story!)

Sarah's sleep journey

Our first daughter, Beth, was born in 2011 and, from day one, I was determined to 'get it right' when it came to sleep. I had read lots of books when I was pregnant and was horrified when hearing others' stories of babies that still woke up frequently at one year plus or had developed 'bad' sleep habits and so would not sleep by themselves. This was not to be for me; I had read the books, I knew what to do and was ready with tips for Moses baskets and cot settling. Beth had different ideas.

She would frequently fall asleep on me and then spring awake as soon as I tried to put her down. I tried everything from expensive baby sheepskin-type blankets for her to lie on to rolled-up muslin cloths to help her feel more snug. Nothing seemed to work. She woke up frequently and although she would fall asleep easily again when I fed her, I would lie her down with dread, fearing her eyes springing open as soon she was laid down by herself.

The sleep deprivation was intense and I remember feeling incredibly disempowered as a mother – surely I was doing something wrong … How come everyone else's baby slept and mine didn't? I had lots of advice, from leaving her to cry to giving her food early, none of which seemed to go with my gut instinct, which was that she was waking up because she wanted to be cuddled. It wasn't until she was about five months old that I finally decided to go with what I felt to be right and stopped obsessing about trying to get her to sleep by herself.

When I was pregnant with my second child, I knew that I would feel differently. We didn't even bother trying to get a cot organised as I knew that the baby would be sleeping in with me. Our only concern was trying to ensure a sleeping environment that was safe for mum, dad, toddler and baby. When Arwen arrived, I felt much more chilled out about sleep. I knew how much easier it was going to be for my own well-being if I just followed my gut instinct and since we had been co-sleeping with Beth for two years, I had gathered a lot of knowledge on the benefits of this way of sleeping, as well as how to do it safely. From day one, Arwen has slept in with me. She takes her naps in the sling (an essential when running around after a busy toddler!) and we follow her sleeping cues entirely. She has never had to be in a sleeping environment by herself, and – no surprise here really – we have had no sleep issues at all. She wakes up a couple of times in the night to feed and as I am right there, she never has to cry to get my attention. No one else even wakes up and she often drops straight back off to sleep with her little hand reassuringly touching me. I feel a bit guilty now when people speak of the inevitable sleep deprivation that comes with new babies – not in this house! We all get a decent night's sleep with no issues so far (four months in).

When I think about where I was at when Beth was four months old, the difference could not be more stark. At that point, I had decided it was too dangerous for me to drive in the daytime as I felt so spaced out. Who knows whether it is just because Arwen sleeps better than Beth did at that age. Or is it because we are so much more relaxed about sleep this time around. Or a combination of the two. I feel that it must make a difference that she has never had to wake up and crave the warmth of a cuddle. Oh, and we still haven't needed that Moses basket!

Chapter 4

The effect of diet on sleep

Have you ever noticed the effect upon your sleep of what you eat and drink, from the drowsy feeling brought about by eating a large Sunday lunch, to the buzz caused by caffeine? Most parents are aware of the stimulating effects of too much sugar and artificial colours and flavourings upon their toddlers, while the 'milk drunk' look of a baby full from a feed is one of the most wonderful sights of babyhood. For some reason though, the effects of diet on sleep are rarely discussed in child sleep books or in advice given by experts. The only times food is generally mentioned in relation to sleep is when dream-feeding, weaning onto solids and topping up with formula milk for babies are discussed.

This chapter looks at how our children's diet can affect their sleep. I start by examining how sleep differs between breastfed and formula-fed babies and consider if dream-feeding and weaning onto solids have a positive impact on sleep. I then examine the foods that may encourage sleep, and those that may hinder it, before ending on the issue of food allergies and intolerances. If your child is well out of babyhood already, then skip straight to the section on foods that may help and hinder sleep.

Do breastfed and formula-fed babies sleep differently?

I would like to start by saying I am supportive of all parenting choices, including how you choose to feed your baby. When I talk about the differences between the sleep of formula-fed and breastfed infants I am doing so only because how you feed your child undoubtedly affects their sleep and I think it is important to know what is 'normal' for the way in which you feed your child.

Breast milk is incredibly easy to digest and babies have small stomachs, meaning that the human infant is meant to feed regularly. Breast milk takes around 1½ hours for a baby to digest. Formula milk takes around 3½ hours for a baby to digest. That's a pretty big difference! Why is this? Human breast milk provides just the right balance of nutrients for a baby, comprising well over 200 different ingredients, and the composition continually changes, depending upon the baby's needs. Breast milk is higher in carbohydrate (lactose), but lower in protein than formula milk. The protein in breast milk is also different to that found in formula milk and is more easily digested, as well as providing immune-boosting properties. Breast milk contains approximately 4 per cent fat, 1 per cent protein and 7 per cent carbohydrate (mostly lactose), and contains around 70 calories per 100ml.[1] In comparison, formula milk contains around 3.5 per cent fat, 3.5 per cent protein and 5 per cent carbohydrate, and around 80 calories per 100ml. It is this different balance of nutrients that makes it harder for a baby to digest formula milk.

Another important difference between formula milk and breast milk is the composition of the protein found in the milk. The protein in milk is comprised of casein (what some people call 'curds', as they form into rubbery curds in the stomach) and whey (which remains in a liquid form in the stomach). Breast milk is comprised of around 30 per cent curds and 70 per cent whey, meaning that the large majority of it passes quickly through the digestive system, as it doesn't curdle into the component that is harder to digest. Cow's milk, however, contains around 80 per cent curds and 20 per cent whey. Baby calves have very different needs and are much more independent than baby humans, who are meant to stay close to their mothers and feed regularly, hence the biological difference in the two milks. Most formula manufacturers artificially manipulate the whey and curd ratio to try to mimic that of breast milk and science is finding more sophisticated ways of doing so. It is important to understand, however, that formula manufacturers are trying to create this ratio from a milk intended for a different species, therefore its natural composition is vastly different to that of human breast milk. The effects of an artificially manipulated product will never quite be the same as the natural version and, despite the advances of science, it is reasonable to expect a difference in the way in which breast milk and formula milk are digested. This difference obviously has an impact on the frequency of feeds needed by the baby, and it is reasonable to expect a breastfed baby to need to feed more regularly, both during the daytime and night. This frequent feeding enhances the protective effect of breastfeeding, both on the baby's developing immune system and in their susceptibility to cot death (SIDS). Formula-fed babies are at an increased risk of SIDS compared to those who are breastfed. Research in 2009 found that, at one month of age, babies who were not exclusively breastfed had double the risk of dying from SIDS, compared to babies who were exclusively breastfed, and this significant protective effect was not seen in babies who were mixed- or combination-fed.[2] In other words, for an otherwise exclusively breastfed baby, giving just one bottle of formula at night can put them at a higher risk of SIDS.

Will giving a bottle of formula at night help a baby to sleep through the night?

I have heard this advice many times, not just from well-meaning friends and relatives, but also from medical professionals too, including GPs and health visitors, which makes it even more worrying when you find out that it is completely false. When you think about the differences in the make-up of breast milk and formula milk it appears logical that babies who are formula-fed will wake less at night, as their tummies stay fuller for longer because of the harder-to-digest milk. However, this is a naïve assumption, as it presumes that babies only wake at night because of hunger, which we know from earlier chapters is not true. It is normal for babies to wake at night for any number of reasons, including their underdeveloped circadian rhythms, shorter sleep cycles, more time spent in REM sleep, their natural segmented sleep pattern, the protective effect of spending more time in lighter sleep states, the need to be in close proximity to their parents, discomfort, being too cold or too hot . . . or almost any other reason. I get so frustrated by the current trend of assuming that babies only wake at night because they are hungry, and that filling them up will ensure they sleep all night: they don't and they won't.

Research in 2010 set out to discover whether formula-fed babies and their mothers slept for longer than those who were breastfed. The results may surprise those who believe that formula feeding is the secret to a good night's sleep, as the researchers found no such association. Measuring the sleep of three different groups of mothers – those who were exclusively breastfeeding, those who were formula-feeding and those who were combination-feeding – they found absolutely no difference in terms of the amount or quality of sleep experienced. They concluded that 'women should be told that choosing to formula feed does not equate with improved sleep'.[3]

Another point to bear in mind is the relatively unknown fact that night-time breastfeeding 'ingredients' actually aid sleep. Research in 2012 found that breast milk produced at night contains significant levels of melatonin, the sleep hormone.[4] This makes biological sense, as the mother's melatonin levels will naturally rise in the evenings in harmony with her circadian rhythms, and this melatonin is then passed through her breast milk to her baby; much like her baby sharing her melatonin in utero. If we remember that babies under three months old have no established circadian rhythms we realise how important this clever trick of nature is. As the researchers commented, 'We speculate that melatonin which is supplied to the infant via breast milk plays a role in improving sleep ... in breast-fed infants compared to formula-fed ones.' For babies who are well on their way to establishing their own circadian rhythms, the extra sleep hormones in night-time breast milk are an added benefit.

Melatonin isn't the only sleep hormone contained in breast milk at night; it also contains more tryptophan, another chemical that aids sleep (see page 70).

Night-time breastfeeding also differs from daytime feeding in the quantity produced. As night falls, a mother will produce more prolactin, the hormone which governs the production of breast milk. This means that she will produce more milk at night, which in turn helps to ensure that babies receive all they need throughout the night. It's no surprise then that babies may want to feed more frequently at night when their mother is producing more breast milk.

Do dream-feeds encourage better sleep?

This myth also relies on the assumption that babies only wake at night because they are hungry. We know this isn't true: yes, babies do wake at night because they are hungry, but we mustn't forget how different their sleep is to that of an adult and how normal it is for them to wake frequently at night for all the reasons mentioned previously. The downside of dream-feeding is the risk of unintentionally waking a baby fully while they are mid-way through a sleep cycle, which may create an unhappy, overtired baby who finds it hard to begin a new sleep cycle. What worries me more about dream-feeding, however, is that it may negatively impact on a baby's developing circadian rhythm, causing artificial waking patterns; the chance of overfeeding an otherwise demand-fed baby; and, lastly, creating a reliance on a late-night feed. If your baby naturally stirs at 10 or 11pm for a feed you can pre-empt their crying and catch them as they begin to rouse, which may make it easier to help them settle into another sleep cycle, but if they don't naturally wake at this time I feel that dream-feeds should be avoided, as the potential risks outweigh any potential benefits.

Does weaning a baby onto solids help their sleep?

What is this obsession with feeding babies to make them sleep? No sooner have we grown out of the dream-feeding and giving-a-night-time-bottle-of-formula-milk recommendations than we are hit with another – that of weaning a baby onto solids to make them sleep through the night. Again, this is a myth that ignores the norms of infant sleep and the reasons behind frequent night wakings. In many cases a baby's sleep regresses after they are weaned onto solids, particularly if this is done too early. This can cause digestive reactions to the new solid food, the most common of these being constipation. Another thing to bear in mind about the introduction of solids is that sometimes a baby's daytime milk intake tails off dramatically due to eating solids during the daytime and they may want to catch up on milk feeds during the night.

Scientific research doesn't support the idea that weaning a baby onto solid foods will help them sleep through the night. Research has consistently found no difference in the sleeping habits of babies who had been weaned onto solids or were given baby rice prior to bedtime.[5] Weaning before six months of age carries several risks for babies, including an increased risk of asthma, eczema, allergies and digestive problems.[6] Bear these risks in mind and don't be tempted to try to wean your baby early in an attempt to get more sleep, particularly given the evidence showing it makes no difference.

Does eating a banana before bedtime help a child to sleep through the night?

Have you heard this one? It seems to have become popular in the last few years, but, like most other sleep advice, there is no evidence that it works. There are, however, certain foods that can encourage a better night's sleep, particularly those foods that are high in a chemical known as tryptophan. Tryptophan is an amino acid and an essential part of the human diet because our bodies are unable to make it, and the only way we can get enough is through our diet – although, as I mentioned earlier, it is a constituent of breast milk. Tryptophan is an important component in the manufacture of serotonin and melatonin, the hormone of sleep, and for this reason many suggest that foods containing high levels of tryptophan may help us to sleep. Research, however, has found that although increased tryptophan intake augmented feelings of sleepiness it doesn't decrease the amount of night wakings.[7] Tryptophan is a component of most protein-based foods such as meat, cheese, eggs, fish and poultry. Of commonly eaten food items, the highest levels of tryptophan can be found in Parmesan and Cheddar cheese, chicken and turkey, sunflower and sesame seeds, lamb, beef and salmon, all of which contain over 0.2 grams of tryptophan per 100 grams of food. Bananas, on the other hand, contain only 0.01 grams of tryptophan per 100 grams, so are a relatively poor source of tryptophan in comparison to most other commonly eaten food items. If bananas do anything to help sleep, it is probably due to nothing more than the child being hungry or a simple placebo effect.

Are there any foods that can cause sleep problems?

There are a number of substances that are consistently linked to sleep problems in children, namely artificial colourings, artificial flavourings, caffeine and monosodium glutamate.

Removing artificial colourings, especially tartrazine, from a child's diet has repeatedly been shown to reduce sleep disturbances. Tartrazine, also known as E102, is a very common food colouring, used mainly to colour foods yellow. It can often be found in ice cream, ice lollies, jelly, crisps, breakfast cereals, biscuits, fruit cordials and many different sweets; alarmingly, it is also commonly found in children's medications. Research conducted in 1994 at a children's hospital in Australia found that 'restlessness, and sleep disturbance are associated with the ingestion of tartrazine in some children'.[8] This echoed findings of earlier research, which found an increase in time taken to go to sleep at night, as well as night awakenings.[9]

Another set of substances, known as salicylates, may also negatively affect child sleep. Salicylates occur naturally in plants, including apples, oranges, peanuts, red grapes and tomatoes.

Salicylates are also found in cocoa beans, which are used to make chocolate. Unfortunately, scientific evidence of a link between salicylates and sleep is scant, with only one very small study conducted in the late 1970s showing a link between salicylate ingestion and sleep disturbances in children.[10] Anecdotally, however, many swear that their child's sleep is negatively affected by salicylate ingestion and that improvements occurred when it was removed from their child's diet. Note that any such changes to a child's diet should only be made in consultation with a medical professional.

Many parents report that too much sugar makes their children hyperactive and has a negative impact on their sleep. This is certainly something I noticed in my own children. Considering that the last food of the day eaten by many children is a dessert after their evening meal, this could be very pertinent to sleep; even more so when you consider that it is often a chocolate-based dessert that is not only full of sugar and contains salicylates, but also caffeine, a known stimulant. I would suggest limiting sugar in your child's diet as much as possible, particularly in the evenings.

Cow's milk protein allergy, lactose intolerance and sleep problems

Many confuse cow's milk protein allergy (CMPA) and lactose intolerance, but they are very different. The key is in the name: an allergy is a (potentially) serious immune system response, whereas an intolerance is the inability to digest a certain substance in food. Another difference is usually seen in the timing of the response after eating the offending food: an allergy usually elicits a fast reaction, whereas an intolerance can manifest several hours later. Allergies occur in response to only a very small amount of the offending ingredient, whereas an intolerance usually means a small amount can be eaten with no ill effects.

Both CMPA and lactose intolerance are fairly common in babies and children. A child usually outgrows both conditions by the age of five, but it is estimated that around one in twenty adults will still suffer from lactose intolerance. Symptoms include diarrhoea, constipation, tummy cramps, wind and bloating, all of which can understandably make a child uncomfortable and lead to disrupted sleep. Unfortunately, despite the common incidence of both conditions, not much research has been conducted into their effects on baby and child sleep but I come across many parents of babies and toddlers suffering from CMPA or lactose intolerance and related sleep problems who report dramatic improvements in sleep after diagnosis and an exclusion diet.

Research looking at babies aged between two and ten months found that after diagnosis of CMPA and subsequent removal of milk protein from their diets, sleep normalised in the participants, with all babies sleeping for longer at night.[11] After reintroducing milk protein into their diets for a week, sleep deteriorated again in all cases. Further research studied the effects of switching the milk intake of infants diagnosed with cow's milk intolerance. For those babies that were breastfed, the mothers adopted a dairy-free diet and for those that were bottle-fed, formula milk was changed to a special hydrolysed prescription. After four weeks, three-quarters of the babies 'achieved a stable sleep pattern within the study period', indicating a correlation between milk intolerance and sleep patterns.[12]

Omega-3 supplements

Recent research has suggested that supplementing a child's diet with omega-3 DHA (long-chain fatty acids usually found in fish and algae) can improve their sleep. In 2014, a team of researchers from the University of Oxford studied the effects of giving a group of children 600mg per day of omega-3 oil over a period of four months. The researchers also measured the levels of omega-3 and omega-6 fatty acids in the children's blood.

The results indicated that those children with low blood levels of omega-3 experienced significantly more sleep problems than children with normal levels. In addition, they discovered that taking the daily supplement of 600mg over a period of four months led to the children having almost an hour's more sleep per night than the children in the control group (those not taking omega-3). The children who received the omega-3 supplement also demonstrated less bedtime resistance and fewer parasomnias (such as night terrors) and night wakings than those in the control group.[13]

There are many omega-3 supplements aimed at babies and children, including liquid-based ones rather than capsules. When selecting a supplement be mindful of the additives included, as many contain artificial sweeteners, colourants and flavourings which could negate the positive effects.

While I believe that diet can and does play a big role in the sleep of children under five, I think it is also important to remember that babies and young children naturally sleep 'badly' and we shouldn't rush to pathologise it. If you do suspect that your child is suffering from an allergy or intolerance, however, it is always worth visiting a lactation consultant, a dietician or your GP. Please don't try an exclusion diet without first consulting somebody suitably qualified.

Chapter 5

The problems with modern sleep-training techniques

You just need to leave him to cry a bit; if you keep going to him he'll never learn to self-settle.

Make her a sticker chart and, each morning, if she's been good and slept well, give her a sticker. When the chart is full up she can have a special reward for being such a good girl.

Don't make eye contact, don't have a conversation, just take him straight back to his room and firmly say 'It's bedtime now', he'll soon learn.

Make sure you give her lots of praise for staying in her own bed all night, tell her what a 'good girl she is' and make a big fuss of 'how grown up she is now'.

Never let a baby fall asleep on the breast or in your arms, they must always be put down awake. They might protest a bit, but it's for the best. You don't want to make a rod for your own back.

Pick up your baby if they cry, the minute they calm down put them back down again, if they cry pick them up again, but put them straight back down again when they stop. They need to learn to fall asleep alone.

Put your child in bed, then leave the room and close the door; if they cry go back in and tell them 'it's bedtime' and leave again, do this as often as you need, but don't cuddle them or say anything else.

Put him in his cot and walk out, if he cries in distress or pain go to him; if he's just protesting then leave him, even if he vomits – actually especially if he vomits as he'll only be doing that for attention. He can't learn that if he vomits you'll pick him up!

Sit at the side of your baby's cot and hold their hand, but don't pick them up. Try to move further away from them each night until there is some distance between you and the cot until finally you're outside the room.

Put her to bed and sit next to her but completely ignore her. This is gentle because you're not leaving her alone. Eventually she will fall asleep.

Buy a special sleep trainer clock that provides a visual clue for your child to know what is an acceptable time to get up. That way he'll know whether he's allowed to get up or not just by looking at the clock. If the clock says no he knows he has to stay in bed for longer.

I could go on almost indefinitely. How many of these gems have you heard? Quite a few I would imagine. As far as I'm concerned, not one of these tips is gentle. I believe that every single one of these sleep-training methods is disrespectful to the child and, in most cases, even if it gets the desired result initially, the effect is often short-lived.

As a parent, what are your long-term goals for your relationship with your child? What sort of person would you like them to become? What sort of qualities would you like them to have? The following are really important to me; perhaps they are to you, too?

- I want to have a close relationship with my child, not just now, but in the future, when they're adults.

- I want my child to trust me, to know that they can tell me anything and come to me with any problem and know that I'll always be there for them.

- I want my child to know that I love them unconditionally – and always will.

- I want my child to know that I respect them, that their needs – both physical and emotional – matter to me.

- I want my child to know that their well-being is paramount to me. I will do everything I can to help them to grow up healthy and happy.

- I want my child to be confident and independent.

- I want my child to grow to have empathy; to value others' feelings as much as their own.

- I want my child to be kind to themself and to others. I want them to be thoughtful.

- I want my child to be trusting of others, and to be trustworthy.

- I want my child to be secure and happy and be able to form a good relationship with their future partner.

Now I want to look at some of those sleep-training suggestions I listed at the beginning of the chapter and how they fit with your parenting goals, and I don't just mean the short-term goal of 'getting a good night's sleep for the first time in ages'.

The downsides of typical sleep-training techniques

Controlled crying

Let's start with controlled crying and 'cry it out'. Does this teach our child that we will always be there for them? Does it teach them that they can rely on us to meet their emotional, as well as physical, needs? Does it teach them that we respect them and their feelings? Does it teach them empathy? Are we being empathic? Does it teach them to be happy and secure and independent by leaving them alone? I don't think so.

I think all we are teaching them is that 'Mummy and Daddy care about your needs between 7am and 7pm, but not between 7pm and 7am'. I know that's simplistic and that wouldn't be your intention, but think of it from your child's point of view: how will they perceive your actions and the intention behind them, especially given their immature brain and inability to think rationally, like an adult? Imagine how confusing it would be for your child. As an analogy, imagine if your partner was only kind, empathic and respectful towards you for 50 per cent of your time together. Would you feel that you could really trust them and rely on them? Of course not. Is this *really* the message you want to give to your child?

Pick up/put down, rapid return and gradual withdrawal

How about picking them up and putting them down, returning to their room rapidly when they cry but not giving them what they really want (your full presence – physically and emotionally), or moving a chair further away from their cot or bed each night. These are all methods commonly touted as 'gentle alternatives to controlled crying and cry it out'. They aren't really gentle though. Do these methods meet your long-term parenting goals? If you use these methods are you respecting your child's needs? Are you giving them the message that you will always be there for them? Are you forging a strong, trustworthy relationship with them? Are you helping them to understand that the feelings of others are important? Again, I don't think so. This behaviour is that of a Jekyll and Hyde parent – loving, empathic and responsive in the daytime but cold, distant and non-responsive at night. How must that make a child feel? How confusing and distressing.

Sleep trainer clocks

With cute animal faces that open their eyes in the morning, glowing clocks that light up and change colour to signify morning and night, and sweet cartoons showing animals sleeping or playing, these might seem like a gentle solution. But what messages are we subconsciously giving to our children when we use them? 'I will only be there for you at a time that I choose is right'; 'If the clock is asleep it doesn't matter what your needs are, they will have to wait'; or perhaps 'I will decide how much sleep you need, regardless of what your body instinctively knows, I know better about your body than you do'. Again, I'm sure most parents don't intend to give these messages to their child, and buy one of these clocks with incredibly good intentions. Think like a child though: as excited as they are to have their own clock, the excitement will soon wear off when they realise that it dictates when they can and cannot have contact with their parents. It doesn't seem so cute when you think of it like that.

The battle of bedtime – winners versus losers

Imagine there are winners and losers in the 'bedtime battle'. Go through the sleep-training scenarios listed above and imagine that they have all worked. They have all resulted in the desired outcome of the child giving up and going to sleep. Who won? The parent(s)? Hurrah, what a victory; finally a sleeping child, a full night's sleep, an end in sight to this terrible exhaustion, a semblance of normality returning to life. Who lost though? If the parent won, then that surely must mean that the child lost? The child needed something from their parents that wasn't given in every single scenario. They lost – and worse. They lost trust in their parents, they lost a little piece of themselves, not just now but in the future. When we win the bedtime battles we always relegate our child into the position of loser. Is that *really* what you want for your child? Is victory really so sweet when we think of it from our child's perspective? Of course some experts would have you believe this is all for the child's own good; that sleep is the most vital thing and if they don't have enough they will be

ill; that you are giving them a gift by helping them to sleep independently.

The trouble is, as a sleep-deprived parent, you are vulnerable
and, as vulnerable as you are, your child is ten times more so.
The fact is, your child needs you. You need to be your child's
advocate and protector; to protect them at night – indeed, you
are all that they have in the dark, scary nights. The key is finding a solution that meets your needs, emotional and physical,
and the needs of your child. It shouldn't be an 'either/or' solution, as offered by the sleep-training methods with which I began
this chapter. You have needs, your child has needs, and there are
no miracle solutions that meet the needs of both, but there are
gentler ways that are considerate to everybody. This is what the
remaining chapters of this book are about.

The downsides of using rewards and praise to encourage better sleep

What about praising and rewarding your child for sleeping all
night, going to bed nicely or staying in their room? They get
stickers, lots of praise and perhaps even a present if they've done
it enough, surely they're a winner then, right? Surely that doesn't
dent their developing personality? Surely that doesn't go against
your long-term parenting goals? Think again.

What are you really doing when you reward or praise your
child for sleeping as you would like them to? Sure, they get a
pretty sticker, or a new teddy bear, but is that what they really
need? Are you being responsive to their night-time needs? Are
you being respectful of their fear, need to feed or need to be
closer to you for reassurance? Are you being empathic and trying
to understand how they feel, validating their very real worries?

Or are they being trained to suppress their needs, to hide their real feelings from you? How might this affect their relationship with you in the future?

When stickers don't work any more will you have to resort to having to bribe them with endless toys or even cash? Is this really the way to foster an authentic relationship of trust and respect? I don't think it is.

How about the idea of loving your child unconditionally – how does praising and rewarding sleep fit in there? What are you really saying? 'I only really love you when you stay quietly in your room all night and leave me alone' perhaps, or 'I do love you, but I love getting a full night's sleep and not seeing you until morning more'? Conditional love, or at least the perception of it, because I'm sure you don't really love your child conditionally, is the start of a slippery slope of teaching your child that the affections of others can be bargained with and manipulated. It won't be long until they start saying 'If I do this, then what will you do?' or 'What will you give me if I do it?' What about their future; what are you teaching them about close relationships? To love and accept their future partner for all that they are, or that love comes with demands and certain provisos? What are you teaching them about themselves? This is the most important point to me. Despite their initial appeal, with rewards and praise masquerading as 'gentle', 'fun' and 'effective' methods, think about their long-term message.

The myth of self-soothing

It's important to examine the concept of 'self-soothing' or 'self-settling' at this point, and why many experts believe that parents should teach this skill to a baby or young child via sleep training. Self-soothing/settling is better known in the world of psychology as 'emotional self-regulation', which simply means the ability of somebody (baby, child or adult) to regulate their own emotions. For example, if a person is feeling angry they are able to calm themselves down; if they are feeling sad, they are able to cheer themselves up and if they are scared, they are able to remove that fear without the aid of anyone or anything else. This is a big issue. Anyone who has experience of toddlers will know that once they get into full-on tantrum mode it is almost impossible to calm them down, let alone for them to be able to do it themselves. Why is this? Quite simply, it is because babies and young children do not have brains that are developed enough to enable them to do this. The area of the brain responsible for the kind of rational thought necessary for emotional self-regulation is not sophisticated enough for this task until well into a child's fifth year of life! Yes, I did say year and not month.

In short, it is biologically, neurologically and physically impossible for a baby, toddler or even perhaps a pre-schooler to be able to 'self-soothe'. Their brains are too immature. It's like trying to teach a three-month-old baby to walk or a one-year-old to have a full-on conversation with you. We accept the physical and neurological limitations of children in almost every other sense, apart from sleep. What we expect of babies and children when it comes to sleep is, in my opinion, impossible. Just five minutes of studying brain biology shows us that 'self-soothing' is not a skill that can be taught; it is physical development that needs time – just as any other developmental skill a child acquires.

A baby, toddler or pre-schooler who no longer calls out for their parents after a bout of sleep training is not miraculously 'self-soothing' and demonstrating an amazing level of brain development unheard of in a child their age; they are simply not calling out for you because they have learnt the very simple fact that you don't come if they do. That, in a nutshell, is what experts who push the need for 'self-soothing' are really advocating, whether they know it or not. I'm not disagreeing that some babies and children seem to be able to get themselves off to sleep quite easily without adult help, as many do, but it is important to realise that this isn't 'self-soothing', it's just a child who naturally needs less parental input, which is not the same thing.

The irony is that the best way to ensure your child grows up with the ability to self-soothe is to respond to their needs early in life. This allows the brain growth necessary to develop the areas responsible for emotional self-regulation. So, ironically, leaving a baby or child to 'self-soothe' can reduce the likelihood that they will be able to do so when their brain is mature enough. If you want to help your child to have good 'self-soothing' skills you need to respond to their needs now. It really is as simple as that.

There are so many things I could say about common sleep-training methods – their safety, their efficacy (and I will cover this a little in a moment) – but the most important aspects to consider are whether they fit in with our long-term parenting goals, whether we are conveying the type of messages we would really like to convey and, perhaps crucially, we are sacrificing the needs of our child for our own. I think we are putting our child's needs second when we use the methods I listed at the start of this chapter.

The risks of sleep training

Are there any other risks with the common sleep-training methods I have mentioned? The simple answer is 'Yes'. The long answer is more along the lines of 'Yes, there almost definitely are, but the research is just not conclusive enough to categorically state what they are', which is deeply frustrating. Obviously if someone is leaving a child to vomit, we don't need scientific research to prove the dangers. The psychological effects are harder to prove and there is a growing sense of unease among many professionals, as well as parents, about the way babies and young children are treated at night-time.

The Australian Association of Infant Mental Health (AAIMH) has famously issued a 'position' paper on controlled crying, in which it states: 'AAIMH is concerned that the widely practiced technique of controlled crying is not consistent with what infants need for their optimal emotional and psychological health, and may have unintended negative consequences ... Crying is a signal of distress or discomfort from an infant or young child. Although controlled crying can stop children from crying, it may teach children not to seek or expect support when distressed.' They follow this up with, 'The demands of Western lifestyles and some "expert" advice has led to an expectation that all infants and young children should sleep through the night from the early months or even weeks ... Many parents become distressed and exhausted when their infants and young children cry at night, in part because of the physical strain of getting up and going to their babies to re-settle them, and sometimes in part because of the unrealistic expectation that babies "should" sleep through the night.'

A similar position is presented on the Infant Sleep Information Source (ISIS) website, from psychologists at the University of Durham's Sleep Laboratory: 'Almost no research has looked at the processes occurring in babies' brains and bodies during sleep training; we therefore have no way of knowing if a baby or child that is not crying is in fact asleep, or is in what is known as a "dissociative" state (meaning that the baby has "withdrawn" in response to the stress caused by being left alone, with cries not being responded to, and has shut off their normal responses to being alone, i.e. crying). If the baby who has settled following sleep training is indeed asleep, is their sleep "normal" or is it different to that of babies who have not undergone the process?' They summarise thus, 'Overall, there is good evidence that sleep-training methods can change babies' sleep patterns in the short term. What is less clear is how this happens, and what other – unintended – consequences of such training might be.'

To date, little research has been carried out looking at the effects of sleep training babies and children and how the training elicits a response. Perhaps the most well-known piece of research to date was carried out by Professor Wendy Middlemiss in 2012. In her small study of four- to ten-month-olds, Middlemiss set out to investigate whether babies were actually calm when they no longer cried out in the night following sleep training. The research measured the cortisol (stress levels) of both mothers and their children during controlled crying. On day three, most of the babies were 'broken' and no longer cried. This is the point when many people would believe they had created a calm, self-soothing baby. The study results, however, did not indicate this. The cortisol levels of the children were just as elevated as they were during the first two days of crying. So they were quiet, but just as stressed: they hadn't 'self-soothed' at all, instead they were just not communicating their distress to their mothers. The mothers, however, hadn't picked up on their baby's distress hence their stress hormone levels were normal. Professor Middlemiss explains this finding by saying, 'When babies stopped crying during the sleep intervention, the mothers' physical cue to their distress was eliminated. The mothers' response to the apparent absence of infants' distress, was a reduction in her physiological levels of stress. Almost an, ahhh, my baby is okay now ... I can be okay. You can almost imagine the possible relief a mother might feel when sleep had become such a distressing event.' She goes on to say, 'Without communicating this distress to mothers, mothers didn't "see" the indicator of their distress. It seems that in this way, without this behaviour cue in this setting, mothers and infants had a different response to the experience.'[1] This research is not without its flaws, and Professor Middlemiss herself recognises this and is keen for more work to be done, but to date it is the best research we have to indicate what many have instinctively believed for so long. That sleep training does not meet the needs of children.

Is sleep training effective in the long term?

Considering how many people recommend sleep training, particularly those who are medically qualified (such as GPs, health visitors and paediatricians), you'd expect there to be a pile of scientific evidence attesting to its long-term effectiveness. Not so. Alarmingly, although there is a convincing amount of evidence showing that sleep training is effective in the short term, that is weeks to months, this isn't the case in the long term. In fact, most of the research undertaken to prove the safety and efficacy of sleep training clearly shows that, in the long term, sleep training is not effective. In many cases those children who are sleep-trained *regress* in their sleep and have more problems than those who were not sleep-trained. A systematic review published in 2013 agrees, with the authors stating, 'Despite substantial investment in recent years in implementation and evaluation of behavioural interventions for infant sleep in the first 6 months, these strategies have not been shown to decrease infant crying, prevent sleep and behavioural problems in later childhood, or protect against postnatal depression.'[2] This review comprised an extensive search of all studies related to infant sleep training published between 1993 and 2013, leading the authors to conclude that sleep training does 'not decrease infant crying, prevent sleep and behavioural problems in later childhood, or protect against postnatal depression. In addition, behavioural sleep interventions risk unintended outcomes, including increased incidence of problem crying, premature cessation of breastfeeding, worsened maternal anxiety, and, if the infant is required to sleep either day or night in a room separate from the caregiver, an increased risk of Sudden Infant Death Syndrome.'

Research published in 2012 came to the same conclusion regarding the long-term effectiveness (or rather, lack of) of sleep training, with the researchers commenting, 'There was no evidence that ... effectively reduced parent-reported sleep problems and maternal depression during infancy had long-lasting harmful or beneficial effects on child, child–parent, or maternal outcomes by 6 years of age.'[3] In other words, for those who were sleep-trained in the first year of life no long-lasting positive result was seen by the time the child was six years old.

Now, I don't know about you but if I was putting my child through the trauma of sleep training I would at least want to see lasting results a few months, if not years, down the line in exchange for the inherent risks. The idea that in only a few months, or even a year, the child's sleep would be right back where it started would certainly put me off, particularly when you think how detrimental it can be to the child and your long-term parenting goals. This is precisely why I looked for another way with my own children. The remainder of this book is devoted to the method I used. Let's start with BEDTIME – the gentle way to encourage more sleep.

Chapter 6

BEDTIME:
practical sleep tips

Based on my experience as a mother of four, and having worked with thousands of parents of children under five, I have come up with seven points that help young children sleep. That's not to say that all seven will appeal to you and work for your family, but there will be something that will. The key is finding what works best for you. Some children need all seven steps to be implemented for them to sleep as soundly as possible, while others require only one or two. Irrespective of how many you use, it is important that you give each one time to work.

Right at the beginning of this book, I said that there is no miracle solution for getting children to sleep through the night, wake later in the morning, go to bed more easily and nap well during the day. That is true of my approach, too. My BEDTIME suggestions are all gentle, and gentle techniques take time to work. A realistic time to expect noticeable changes is six weeks. Please don't try something once or twice and think 'Oh, that doesn't work', before giving up on it. If you want to make changes in your child's sleep that last you have to be prepared to give the techniques time to work. If you are committed enough there will be something here that helps you. I promise.

Introducing my BEDTIME acronym

Bedsharing and co-sleeping
Expectations
Diet
Transitional objects
IT and screen time
Me-time
Environment

Bedsharing and co-sleeping

In Chapter 3 we looked at the incidence and normality of bedsharing and co-sleeping around the world. Remember that bedsharing is sharing a sleeping surface with your child and co-sleeping is sharing a room with your child. Both of these practices tend to be frowned upon in Western society, where it is believed that children should be independent as soon as possible and allowing them to sleep in the same bed or room as us, particularly after babyhood, will create clingy, damaged children. This is not true.

The emergence of independence is a developmental milestone. It is the very nature of every baby and child to be dependent upon us. In short, they need us to survive and to stay healthy in body and in mind. As a child grows, their brain matures and they become capable of more sophisticated behaviour, including that of being independent, but while they are still tiny – and children under five years old are still tiny – they need us. Time and again researchers and psychologists have shown us that the key to developing a good level of independence in children is to first allow them to be dependent on us. The very word 'independent' implies that one first needs to have been 'dependent' in order to become less so. A child who is allowed to be dependent on his parents has much more chance of growing up to be independent, secure and confident in his own skin. If we force a child to become independent, for fear of him being 'clingy' and laughed at when he 'should be a big boy by now', we risk the very thing we are so keen on him developing and are more likely to create a needy adult. I can't stress this enough: we should *never* be scared of creating clingy children by allowing them to be dependent on us and fulfilling their needs, for fulfilling these needs is the very best way to create confident, independent individuals.

Don't just take my word for it though. Science has proven that sharing a room or a bed with a child throughout the first five years of life is psychologically risk free and most likely beneficial. Research in Switzerland in 2005 found that at the age of four almost 40 per cent of the five hundred children studied were sleeping in their parents' bed at least once a week.[1] Interestingly, they also found that those who slept separately from their parents as a baby were no less likely to share a bed with their parents by the time they reached school age. This highlights the fact that you cannot teach, or 'train', independence by putting a baby to sleep in a separate room from their parents; their need for close contact with their parents remains throughout their childhood.

Science also provides us with proof that sharing a bed with babies, toddlers and pre-schoolers does not cause any psychological damage when they are older. This point is important, since many health professionals and the media frequently warn of the 'clingy and damaged' children that will be created by sharing their parents' beds. In 2002, researchers very clearly found that 'At age 6 years, bedsharing in infancy and early childhood was not associated with sleep problems, sexual pathology, or any other problematic consequences. At age 18 years, bedsharing in infancy and childhood was unrelated to pathology or problematic consequences.'[2] This same research also found that, far from creating problems, bedsharing has a positive effect on the intelligence of children. Researchers commented that 'Bedsharing in early childhood was found to be significantly associated with increased cognitive competence measured at age 6 years.' This isn't the only research that parents who bedshare with their babies, toddlers and pre-schoolers can take comfort from. Research from the USA studied almost one thousand families over a five-year period, collecting data on their sleeping practices. Once the child was five years old their cognitive and behavioural functioning were tested, focusing on their hyperactivity levels and social skills. Unsurprisingly, those children who had regularly bedshared with their parents did not display any more problems than those who had not. Commenting on these results, Dr Lauren Hale, from the University of New York, said 'very little research has investigated the potential developmental consequences of bedsharing during toddler hood. We found that, after adjusting for mother and child characteristics, there were no observed cognitive or behavioural differences between children who bedshare and those who don't. Parents should make decisions about sleeping arrangements based on their specific family circumstances, with the goal of facilitating the best possible sleep for their children.'[3]

If the research proving that bedsharing does not psychologically damage children or make them clingy is not enough to convince the sceptics then perhaps looking at the science that tells us of the benefits of bedsharing into early childhood might? Research in Denmark in 2012 found that bedsharing may decrease a child's risk of obesity in later life. Studying data from over six hundred children, the researchers discovered that those children who had never shared their parents' bed were three times more likely to be overweight compared to those that shared a bed with their parents. Commenting on these results, the lead researcher, Dr Nanna Olsen, said: 'The results may suggest that elements of parental social support or other types of positive psychosocial responses of being allowed to enter parents' bed during night may protect against overweight, whereas types of negative psychosocial responses such as feelings of rejection when not being allowed to enter parents' bed may lead to overweight.'[4]

In many countries around the world it is completely normal for children to share a bed or a room with their parents, particularly in Asia, where research has found that 40 per cent of children in China routinely co-sleep or bedshare with their parents until they are six years old. Scientists found that the prevalence of routine bed sharing and room sharing in Chinese children aged between three and six years old was 21 per cent and 19 per cent respectively.[5] Why in the West are we so scared of allowing our children to be dependent upon us, particularly given the research that proves not only the lack of harm, but the potential benefits and how normal it is around the world? Could sharing a bed or a room help your family perhaps?

I asked some mothers who had chosen to bedshare or co-sleep with their child why they had done so and what they felt was the most important thing they had learnt about child sleep since becoming a parent. Here are some of their answers:

I learned not to stress about where your baby sleeps. I tortured myself during the early weeks trying to get my son to sleep in his Moses basket because I thought that's what I was 'supposed' to do. I guiltily stumbled into bedsharing when my son was three weeks old, but the effect was immediate.

I learned that co-sleeping is the most natural way to sleep with a baby. A baby falling asleep in the mom's warm arm or chest is a complete experience.

I learned that it doesn't matter if they only sleep when they're in bed with me or on my lap. There is no rod for my back and they grow up so fast you should cherish every moment they need you close.

I learned that if my toddler needs me (or my husband) to sit by her bedside while she goes to sleep, or lie with her in the night when she wakes, then that's fine/normal and I'm not going to resort to sleep training as I did briefly with my first child (we all hated it – never again!). I've learned to actually enjoy these times instead of see them as behaviours to be changed through sleep training. (I know she'll grow out of it at some point and when she's older I'll probably miss it!)

I learned that bedsharing is not dangerous in the 'blanket statement' way it was communicated to me through media before I was a parent, and reinforced by health professionals when I was. That is, there are safety guidelines that make it as safe/safer than lone-sleeping, in terms of SIDS.

I learned that provided you pay attention to safety guidelines, co-sleeping is perfectly safe and from a historical point of view ... normal!

I learnt that babies and toddlers quickly grow into children who want and demand independence. Snuggle into those little ones and let them sleep in your arms while you can, it's really a fleeting moment of childhood, gone in the blink of a sleep-deprived eye. (I'm writing that while number four snoozes in my arms, the only one of four that still does, sniff sniff.)

How to bedshare with your child

Although it can be an absolute life-saver for some families, bed-sharing isn't for everyone and it is important that you are comfortable with it if you give it a try. If you like the idea of giving your child a little more reassurance at night, without actually sharing a bed with them, then skip to the co-sleeping section which comes after this.

You may be aware of the media propaganda surrounding the safety of bedsharing. What you may not realise is that most of what you read in newspapers or see in television news reports is a journalist's interpretation of a press release and they are unlikely to have looked at the research or checked the study methodology for flaws or the results for bias and opinions. This means that the general public is presented with inaccurate and possibly scaremongering information. In truth, what we know from the large amount of research into bedsharing is that, if the safety guidelines are followed, it is no more risky than a baby sleeping in a cot.

The first variable to consider when thinking about bedsharing with a child under one, is whether or not the mother is breastfeeding. Bedsharing and breastfeeding work together wonderfully: research indicates that sharing a bed with a baby supports breastfeeding and can help it to continue for longer.[6] We know from research that formula-fed and breastfed babies sleep differently, particularly at two to three months, which is the peak risk period for SIDS.[7] At this stage, formula-fed babies are significantly less arousable than breastfed babies, which could spell disaster for a formula-fed baby who accidentally slips under the covers while sleeping next to their mother. The lowered arousability levels mean they are less likely to wake, and alert their parent that they are in danger, than a breastfed counterpart.

A lesser-known phenomenon is that formula-feeding and

breastfeeding mothers also sleep differently. Breastfeeding mothers appear to be more in tune with their babies during the night compared to mothers who formula-feed. This means they may also be more easily aroused and therefore more likely to awaken if their baby stops breathing, or slips under a blanket. To add to this, breastfeeding mother and baby dyads tend to sleep in a different position to formula-feeding mothers and their babies. Research observing the sleep of mothers and babies sharing a bed at the University of Durham's Parent–Infant Sleep Lab highlights how different these sleeping positions are. Professor Helen Ball, head of the sleep lab, comments on this, saying, 'Current and ex-breastfeeders positioned their babies and themselves in different ways from and were oriented towards their babies for much more of the night than mothers who had never breastfed. The physical relationship between mum and baby in the bed was different. Never-breastfeeders had a face-to-face relationship, positioning their babies at face height in the bed. Breastfeeders, whether currently breastfeeding or not, had a baby-to-breast relationship, positioning their baby at breast height, curling up around them for sleep, and creating a space with their bodies for the baby to sleep in. Never-breastfeeders slept side by side, and spent much more time facing away from one another, sometimes even turning their backs.' For all of these reasons it is important that you only share a bed with your baby if you are breastfeeding. If your baby is formula-fed they should always have their own sleep surface. For toddlers and pre-schoolers, who are much more robust and find it easier to alert parents to any problems, this is less important, although all other safety guidelines are just as pertinent.

If you want to try bedsharing you must follow these safety guidelines.

BEDSHARING SAFETY GUIDELINES

- Only share a bed with your baby if the baby is breastfed. Babies who are formula-fed should have their own sleep space.

- Both parents should be non-smokers and, importantly, the mother also should not have smoked during pregnancy.

- Both parents should not have consumed any alcohol.

- Both parents should not have taken any recreational or prescription drugs.

- Parents should not be 'excessively tired', based on their own instinct, although some suggest they should not have had less than five hours' sleep in the last twenty-four hours.

- The mother should always sleep between her partner and the baby; the baby should never be in the middle of the bed. This is also true for any older siblings.

- The sleeping surface should be firm (no memory foam) and designed for sleep: this means a bed only; never sleep with a baby on a sofa, hammock or beanbag.

- Prevent the baby from rolling onto the floor; many parents decide to sleep on a mattress on the floor to prevent this from happening.

- Keep pillows well away from the baby. The baby should sleep at the same level as the mother's breasts, not her head.

- The mother should lie on her side and form a protective frame around her baby (see illustration below).

- Keep duvets and blankets away from the baby to prevent risk of smothering and to ensure the baby does not overheat. (Some mothers wear onesies and thick dressing gowns to bed to keep themselves warm.)

- Tie long hair back and do not wear nightclothes with loose ties in order to prevent accidental strangulation.

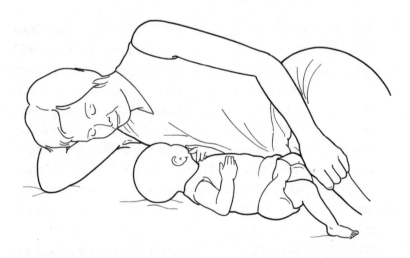

Using a side-car crib

Many parents love the idea of sleeping next to their baby but are sometimes worried about sticking to the safety guidelines. Some are not keen on sharing their bed space, perhaps if their bed is not big enough, and others should not sleep in the same bed as their baby for safety reasons (these include if the baby is formula-fed, is very small for their age or premature and if the mother is significantly overweight). Sometimes parents already have an older child in their bed when a new baby arrives and decide to continue sharing with their older child and put the baby in a side-car crib.

There are many specially designed side-car cribs available (see page 281). These special cribs fix to the bed in the most secure and safe way possible and allow for instant access and close prox-imity to the baby, while providing parents with extra security and peace of mind.

Moving your baby out of your bed

Many parents are concerned that if they allow their baby into their bed they will be creating a rod for their own back and will never get their child to leave. Rest assured, your child will soon be independent enough to move of their own accord, often at around three to four years of age, but many babies happily move to their own bed much earlier than this. If you are not keen on sharing a bed with a toddler or pre-schooler, a good age to move a baby to their own bed is around six to eight months, when they have passed the fourth trimester and the four- and five-month sleep regression but not yet hit the separation anxiety stage.

My preference would be to allow the child to make the deci-sion, as only then will you know that their needs are met. However, if long-term bedsharing is not for you, make the move as gently and gradually as possible. This could take the form of a cot placed next to you, or, if they are older, a mattress on the floor next to your own bed. Some parents are happy to continue to share their room with their child, in which case there is no need to make any other change. Soon enough your child will want their own space. If you would prefer to move your child into their own room then you can gently encourage them using some of the techniques I suggest in the next section. I can promise you that your child won't want to sleep with you for ever!

How to co-sleep with your child

Co-sleeping with your child means 'rooming in' with them, but with them in their own bed. For some families this isn't viable due to a lack of space in the bedroom, but for others it works really well, particularly with toddlers and pre-schoolers, especially those feeling insecure due to the arrival of a new sibling, starting daycare or experiencing nightmares. Rooming-in offers the best of both worlds: parents have their bed to themselves and the child gets the comfort of sleeping in close proximity to their parents. Some families move a single mattress into the room for the child, while others prefer to buy specially made toddler beds that take up far less space. The added benefit of this is that when the time comes for your child to move to their own room, their bed will already be familiar and comforting to them, making the move far less of a transition.

Co-sleeping can also work especially well for children who have recently become a new big brother or sister. Toddlers and pre-schoolers' sleep can regress after the arrival of a new baby, often because they feel pushed out and unsure of their place in their parents' affections. This can be worsened by the presence of the baby in the parents' bedroom. Inviting the child to share a 'family bedroom' can help them to feel included and more secure, which not only has a positive impact on their sleep, but can also help with their daytime behaviour.

Moving your child out of your room

My preference, when it comes to moving a child to their own bedroom, is to wait until the child is ready. If the transition is child-led then it will almost always go more smoothly. Don't be tempted to move your child out of your room shortly before or after the arrival of a new baby, as this is a time when they need to feel close to you and be reassured of your presence and love. In this scenario, begin the transition to their own bedroom either very early in the pregnancy or a few months after the baby has arrived, when everything has settled down. Also, don't be tempted to encourage your child to move 'because you're a big girl now'. Most young children who have become a big brother or sister struggle with conflicting feelings of wanting to be big and wanting to be little. The 'wanting to be little' feelings can often win out with a new baby in the house, so encouraging them to 'be a big girl' can be counterproductive. Why would they want to be big when it seems like only little children get all the cuddles and attention?

Gentle ways to encourage your child to sleep in their own bedroom include allowing them to decide how it is decorated, what bedding they will have, how the room is set out and filling it with items that are familiar and reassuring for them. Perhaps the most successful encouragement is spending time together in their bedroom in the daytime. It tends to be quite rare that parents do this, yet, if they don't, how will the child build good associations with the room and feel safe and comfortable enough to sleep alone in it? It is vital that you spend at least half an hour every day playing *together* in the child's bedroom. Cuddle and read stories on their bed, play games, listen to music and do jigsaw puzzles; whatever it is that you like to do together that makes your child happy. They must see their bedroom as a happy place, full of good memories and associations, not just a room they are left alone in at night-time. I can't emphasise enough how important it is for you to do this. It is also vital that you never punish your child in their bedroom, by using it for time out or the like, as this will build bad associations that will mean that they are less happy to spend time alone in there at night.

But what about sex?

If bedsharing or co-sleeping is mentioned in the media I can almost guarantee that the journalist or presenter will raise the question 'but how do you stay intimate with your partner with a child in the room?', quickly followed by an expert adding that 'co-sleeping kills relationships'.

Do you know what really kills relationships? Not communicating, taking each other for granted and being exhausted. The simple fact of the matter is that, for the vast majority, having children means a dramatic change to your sex life. Post-birth, mothers not only have to deal with the massive hormonal changes occurring in their body, but they have to adjust to their new postnatal bodies, including swollen and tender breasts, stretch marks and saggy tummies, and some have to also deal with scars to their perineum or bikini lines. All of this can lead mothers to lose interest in sex, at least for a while. Furthermore, adjusting to the new role of parenting and what a huge life change it is, for men as well as women, and libidos tend to take a nose dive wherever the child is sleeping.

Most parents of young children suffer from exhaustion, not just from the sleepless nights, but also from the constant physical demands of changing nappies, feeding, bathing, dressing and tidying up after their child. Again, this often impacts on their sex drive, understandably so. I think acknowledging that sex isn't high on the agenda for most new parents is an important starting point. After this my response is always, if co-sleeping means parents get more sleep and are less exhausted that has to be good for their sex life surely? Less exhausted parents must surely mean more sex? Lastly, is it really true that sex only takes place at night in bed? There are other times and places. It doesn't seem to stop the co-sharing parents in other parts of the world from conceiving a second, third, fourth or fifth child, so they must be doing something, perhaps just not in the bedroom.

Expectations

The second of my seven BEDTIME tips comprises two elements. The first is having realistic expectations of your child's sleep and the second is helping them to form associations and expectations around bedtime, particularly through having a good bedtime routine.

Let's start with forming realistic expectations about your child's sleep. Babies and children under five sleep 'badly', or at least that's how we interpret it. They don't really sleep *badly*, they sleep normally for them.

It infuriates me when people ask 'Is he good?', when what they really mean is 'Does he sleep all night?' Babies and young children aren't 'bad' and to think they are, particularly for waking at night, is ridiculous. Is a child bad because they get hungry every two or three hours through the night? Is a child bad because when they wake at the end of a sleep cycle they feel insecure and want a cuddle from their parents? Is a child really so bad because when they wake after a nightmare, scared, they want our reassurance? Of course not. Adults need to reset their expectations of baby and child sleep and what is normal. Babies and children wake regularly at night, they wake early in the morning, they often don't like to go to bed as early as we want them to, and they take short naps and tend to not take them when we want them to either. These problems are our problems, not our child's.

In the remaining chapters of the book I look at normal sleeping patterns at specific ages, to give you some idea of what to expect from your child's sleep. I explain the reason for these sleeping patterns, as sometimes they are biological and other times they are more psychological in origin. Understanding what your child is experiencing at a certain age means you will be able to empathise with their feelings and the resulting sleep patterns. When you understand what your child is going through, it becomes far easier to make small changes that can have quite a big impact on their night-time sleep and daytime naps.

Helping your child to form good sleep expectations

One of the key ways you can help your child to nap more easily during the day and to sleep better at night is by helping them to form associations and expectations around bedtime. When a child knows what to expect they feel more secure, whether you are setting boundaries for their behaviour, helping them to understand the rhythms of the day or what is and isn't expected of them in different scenarios. One massive difference between adults and children is our ability to tell the time. Young children are almost solely reliant on the setting and rising of the sun to tell them whether it is day or night. They have natural instincts, just like us, but from the moment they are born their parents begin to override these. For those babies put on a feeding schedule, the parent decides whether they should feed or not, regardless of whether they are feeling hungry. For those on a sleeping schedule, the same is true in relation to sleep. Even if feeding and sleeping have been baby-led it is quite rare that they remain toddler- or child-led in the later years. How can we expect our babies and children to recognise their own bodily signs of tiredness if we don't pay attention to them? As a parent, understanding the early signs that your child is tired can be a game changer, as you can then help them to nap or sleep at night before they reach the fractious, overtired stage when they are difficult to calm.

Do you know all of your child's early sleep signs? Here are some typical ones.

Typical signs of tiredness

- Rubbing eyes and yawning

- Red-rimmed, watery eyes

- A glazed look, eyes not focusing

- Ear pulling

- Touching the head repeatedly

- Gaze aversion (not making eye contact with you)

- Increased tantrums

- Increased crying

- Child losing patience/interest in things

- Falling over/being clumsy

Setting a bedtime routine

Young children like to know what to expect so having a good bedtime routine is essential. I don't mean a routine that is set by the clock, with rigid sleep and wake times, but a routine that helps the child to know that nap time or bedtime is approaching.

If you think about your daily routine there are likely to be external triggers that help you to know that bedtime is approaching; perhaps the theme tune to a television programme like the 10 o'clock news, the street lights turning off outside your window or curling up on the sofa after dinner. Similarly, there are often familiar triggers in the morning that signal it's time to get up: birds singing in the garden, or the sound of pipes coming to life as the central heating system comes on. Of course we don't need these triggers to know whether it is time for us to sleep or wake, as we can tell the time, we know when it's getting late and we should be considering going to sleep, or we know when we have half an hour until we must get out of bed. Babies and young children don't and this lack of routine in their lives can be unsettling, as they literally don't know if they are coming or going.

A good nap-time or bedtime routine can have a profound effect on a child's sleep. Research conducted in 2009 looked at the sleep patterns of over four hundred children between the ages of seven months and three years. Half of the group were instructed to implement a simple bedtime routine that consisted of bathing, followed by applying a lotion to the child's skin and then up to twenty minutes of quiet time (which could take the form of a lullaby, bedtime story or cuddles and a quiet chat before bed). The remaining half were told to follow their usual bedtime patterns. After three weeks, parents were asked about their child's sleeping patterns. Those who had consistently followed the bedtime routine every night reported significantly fewer night wakings and found it easier to get their child to sleep. An added benefit was that the mothers in the bedtime routine group also felt that there had been a positive effect on their own mood. This led the researchers to conclude that 'These results suggest that instituting a consistent nightly bedtime routine, in and of itself, is beneficial in improving multiple aspects of infant and toddler sleep, especially wakefulness after sleep onset and sleep continuity, as well as maternal mood.'[8]

I don't think bathing your baby or child every night is necessary, or particularly good for their skin, especially if it is prone to dryness. However, doing a short massage every night is feasible. I use an unscented natural organic edible oil, such as sunflower, for under-threes and a natural lavender or chamomile-based oil (see page 281 for recommendations). Follow this with changing into pyjamas for story time and cuddles, preferably in a darkened room to ensure the best night's sleep possible. A bedtime routine should last somewhere between twenty minutes and half an hour before you expect the child to lie down and go to sleep. This routine not only helps a child to recognise that bedtime is approaching, it also provides valuable one-to-one time for parent and child to connect each evening. This is really important if the child is in daycare or has recently become a big brother or sister. In such cases, if possible, bedtime routines should always be done one child at a time, not in tandem.

Nap-time routines

While research has only focused on the impact of bedtime routines for night-time, they are equally useful for daytime naps. A daytime nap routine may consist of having a snack or some milk, followed by cuddles or a story in the bedroom and perhaps singing a special nap-time lullaby together, choosing a cuddly toy and closing the curtains – always done in the same order, every day.

For both bedtime and nap-time routines don't expect miracles. As with any gentle technique, these will take time to work. The research into bedtime routines studied the effects after three weeks of consistently implementing the routine every night. Try implementing the routines for at least one month before assessing progress. Don't be disheartened if you still don't notice any changes after a couple of weeks: stick with it!

The benefits of story time before bed

As I've already mentioned, one of the benefits of a consistent bedtime routine is the opportunity to connect with your child, one-to-one. It also helps both parent and child to calm down and unwind after a busy day. Storytelling forms a vital part of sleep-time routines in my opinion, yet this has been ousted by TV 'bedtime hour' shows, story CDs and electronic storytellers, which is a shame. Hearing stories is a wonderful way to trigger a child's imagination and to leave them with fantastical happy thoughts as they drift off to sleep. Parents, on the other hand, get to relive childhood favourites and reminisce about the stories they loved as a child. There are other benefits of story time too, not least a proven link between listening to bedtime stories and better sleep.

Research in 2011, looking at over 4,000 families with children up to age five, found that regular bedtime stories not only help to increase the total duration of a child's sleep, but also help them to develop intellectually and reduce bad behaviour. The researchers commented that, 'This research suggests regular use of language-based bedtime routines including singing, reading, and storytelling at bedtime may have a lasting positive benefit for children's sleep duration and cognitive development.'[9] Bedtime stories needn't be long – there are plenty of books featuring stories that are just a page or two long.

Have you ever wondered why your child insists on you reading the same book over and over again? Isn't it infuriating? To a child, though, hearing the same story every day is reassuring; they like to know what happens in the story and they like to be able to tell you what comes next. This goes back to how children need a predictable routine in order to feel safe and secure, especially when it comes to sleep. So, despite the annoyance of reading the same book for the hundredth time, you can smile in the knowledge that however boring it is for you, it is helping your child to sleep. On page 282 you will find some suggestions for books that I think really help children to relax and sleep.

WEEKEND LIE-INS AND STAYING UP LATER

When it comes to expectations and routines, the key is consistency; keeping each and every day the same wherever possible – and that means weekends, too. I know there's a huge temptation to try to encourage a later morning start by having a later bedtime on a Friday or Saturday night, but this is normally counterproductive. Most children won't wake up later if they go to bed later. They usually still wake at the same time, just significantly more grumpy. Moreover, research conducted in 2012 highlights the importance of keeping wake and sleep times consistent across weekdays and weekends. After studying the sleep habits of almost two hundred children, the researchers concluded that 'To encourage earlier bedtimes in children, it is important to take the mother's sleeping and living habits into account and to maintain a regular wake-up and bedtime schedule across weekdays and weekends.'[10] I think the same is true of holidays, too: as ever, consistency is key.

Diet

I have already covered diet at some length in Chapter 5, but there are three important points to bear in mind here. First, it is important to recognise that breastfed babies and formula-fed babies do sleep differently, therefore you need to accept what is normal for your child, depending on how they are fed.

Second, it is important to understand that babies do need night feeds, usually long after most baby 'experts' say that they do. I am not of the opinion that babies should not need feeding in the night after six months, as many experts insist. Some babies need feeding in the night long into their second year of life and, really, the only person who can tell if this is necessary is your baby. There is nothing wrong with your baby if they still need a feed at night, especially if they are breastfed. In chapters 11 to 13 I'll cover some night-weaning suggestions.

The last consideration is what your child is eating and how it may be affecting their sleep, from allergies and intolerances through to foods that can inhibit – and foods that may potentially help – sleep. I examine this in later chapters but do bear in mind that it is always worth considering the impact of your child's diet on their sleep.

Transitional objects

This is just a posh psychological term for comfort objects, comforters or loveys. The term 'transitional object' was coined by the English psychotherapist Donald Winnicott in 1951, at the same time as he introduced the concept of the 'good enough mother' and the two concepts are linked. Put simply, the 'good enough mother' is one who allows her child to attach, or be dependent on her, when he needs to and then to become independent, or detach from her, when he needs to. This process of independence occurs often through accidental moments of separation where the child must learn to be away from the mother. Or as, Winnicott says, 'the good enough mother is one who makes active adaptation to the infant's needs, an active adaptation that gradually lessens according to the infant's growing ability to account for failure of adaptation and to tolerate the results of frustration'. This wonderful concept takes much of the guilt out of parenting. A mother doesn't have to be perfect; in fact Winnicott says it is her imperfections that allow the child to become independent. She just has to be 'good enough'.

A transitional object is simply an object that allows the child to make the transition to independence from the mother. In a way it is like a metaphorical bridge between dependence and independence that allows the child to separate from his mother while still retaining a piece of her in his grasp. This 'piece of the mother' takes the form of a teddy, muslin, blanket or similar that he associates with his mother. Of course, in order for the child to associate an object with his mother, it must first be conditioned so that there is a strong association between the object and the mother (see below). A natural transitional object would be a piece of clothing a mother wears often, such as a dressing gown or even a bra. Children will associate this with their mother as it will have her scent.

It is vital that the transitional object is chosen by the child. This is tough, as invariably they ignore the beautiful teddies and blankets bought by close friends or knitted by Grandma and plump for a grotty old muslin or something similar. If your child has already chosen their transitional object do not take it away from them or try to change it. As Winnicott says, 'It must never change, unless changed by the infant.' Bear in mind, too, that Winnicott believed that only around 60 per cent of babies and young children will take to a transitional object. I have often found that those who are breastfeeding and bedsharing are the ones least likely to want a transitional object.

How to condition a transitional (comfort) object

- If your child already has an object that comforts them don't try to persuade them to use something else.

- If they don't yet have one it is important that you let your child choose what they want to use, irrespective of how you feel about it!

- Begin to condition the transitional object by including it in any activities you do with your child. Snuggle it between you during feeding and cuddling. Tuck it into bed with the two of you, involve it in play and so on.

- Allow at least one month of continuous daily conditioning of the comfort object before deciding if it is having an effect.

- When the comfort object is conditioned don't immediately try to replace yourself with it, but do it gradually.

- Avoid washing the comfort object, as part of the point is that it retains your scent. If you do wash it, expect your child to be unhappy and to spend time re-conditioning it.

- This point probably should have come first, but consider having two comfort objects, exactly the same (equally conditioned), because I speak from first-hand experience when I say how traumatic it is if your child loses theirs.

Another crucial point is that comforters must be easily accessible to the child, at any time of day or night, and they should not need your help to find and hold it. Research carried out in 2004 looked at the ease of access of comforters and concluded, 'Of the children using the comforters classified as "easy access" (i.e. comforters they were more likely to find and hold), 71% were sleeping through the night at 6 months old. The associations were incremental in that of those children who used both "easy access" comforters and comforters requiring parental input, 48% were sleeping through the night at 6 months, and of those children using only parental input comforters only 38% were sleeping through the night.'[11] I think 71 per cent of children sleeping through at six months is highly ambitious. The trial was small, with just over one hundred families studied, and the researchers also do not define what they mean by 'sleeping through' (most medical experts define it as sleeping for a period of five hours), but the difference in ease of access to the comforter still remains despite these limitations.

It is perfectly normal, and very common, for a child to use their comfort object well beyond their fifth year. I know adults who still have one. Is there ever a time when children should stop using one? When it becomes 'too babyish'? I don't think so; as long as your child is deriving comfort from it, who are we to say it is time for them to give it up?

IT – or screen time

I have already covered this topic in Chapter 2, but the impact of screen time cannot be overemphasised. The use of screens can affect sleep negatively in two ways. The first is the impact of the blue/white light source that is emitted, which we know influences the production of melatonin, the sleep hormone. The second is the stimulating effect that television, games and apps can have on the brain, particularly those of young children. Screen time should be limited for everybody, but I'm not saying it is always bad. In very limited doses I think it's OK, particularly when used for educational purposes, but almost every child in Western society spends too much time looking at screens.

Try to make sure that your child has no screen time for the last two hours before bedtime – none at all, and that includes television programmes intended for their age group. In addition, try to reduce screen time during the day, as it can also disrupt circadian rhythms and stimulate the brain, making it harder for children to sleep at night. The basic rule is to keep screen time at an absolute minimum wherever possible and never allow a child to have a television or other screen in their bedroom.

Me-time

You may be wondering what on earth this topic is doing here, because you only get 'me-time' when your child sleeps, and that's why you're so desperate for them to sleep! I promise you there is a point to this, and a very important one at that.

First, as much as your child matters, you matter too. If you run yourself into the ground, who will look after your child? The analogy of the oxygen masks on an aeroplane, so often used by parenting educators, is true. Why do you think the safety briefings tell you to put your oxygen mask on first, before putting it on your children? Every cell in your body would be screaming at you to save your child but what would happen to your child if, in the process of putting on their mask, you lose consciousness and never manage to put your mask on? Who would look after your child then? The same is true for parenting. To look after your child's needs it is imperative you look after your own. You need to eat well, take supplements if necessary, sleep whenever you can (even if that means going to bed at 7pm every night) and treat yourself once in a while to a long bubble bath, a trashy magazine, a box of chocolates, a haircut, a massage, a coffee with friends ... whatever you need to refill your tank every now and again. It also means getting help, asking for help, buying in help if you can afford it or finding free help from support organisa-tions (see Resources, page 279).

There is another relevant point to consider. Research shows that children of mothers who are depressed sleep significantly worse than the children of those who are not. This is a bit of a chicken-and-egg situation. Is it the mother's depression that causes the sleeplessness in the child or the sleeplessness of the child that causes the mother to be depressed? The answer is prob-ably a bit of both; the correlation is strong and a great deal of research has proven the link. In 2014, research found that 'Life stress in the mothers was statistically significant and negatively related to pre-school child's sleep duration.'[12] These findings were echoed by research in 2012: the lead researcher, Dr Douglas Teti, commented, 'We found that mothers with high depressive symp-tom levels are more likely to excessively worry about their infants at night than mothers with low symptom levels, and that such mothers were more likely to seek out their babies at night and spend more time with their infants than mothers with low symp-tom levels. This, in turn, was associated with increased night waking in the infants of depressed mothers, compared to the infants of non-depressed mothers. Especially interesting was that when depressed mothers sought out their infants at night, their infants did not appear to be in need of parental help. They were either sound asleep or perhaps awake, but not distressed.'[13]

Research in 2005 linked sleep deprivation with the onset of depression in mothers, with researchers concluding that 'infant sleep patterns and maternal fatigue are strongly associated with a new onset of depressive symptoms in the post-partum period', which indicates that maternal depression can be worsened by the excessive tiredness caused by sleep deprivation.[14] Research in 2014 highlights a link the other way; in that infants may pick up on their mother's moods and become more distressed as a result. Lead researcher Dr Sarah Waters commented on her findings, saying, 'Our research shows that infants "catch" and embody the physiological residue of their mothers' stressful experiences ... Before infants are verbal and able to express themselves fully, we can overlook how exquisitely attuned they are to the emotional tenor of their caregivers.' She goes on to say, 'Your infant may not be able to tell you that you seem stressed or ask you what is wrong, but our work shows that, as soon as she is in your arms, she is picking up on the bodily responses accompanying your emotional state and immediately begins to feel in her own body your own negative emotion.'[15] This demonstrates the link between maternal mood and child sleep behaviours and highlights why improving our own emotional well-being is a major factor in improving our children's sleep. Taking care of yourself isn't selfish, it is the key to surviving the sleeplessness of early parenting and, quite possibly, the key to solving it too.

Environment

A calming environment is vital in helping your child sleep, and to create it you need to consider how your child's senses are affected by their surroundings.

Lighting

We now know how light influences the production of melatonin (the sleep hormone). Our circadian rhythms are governed by our body's response to the light our eyes perceive. In order to not interrupt your child's body clock with artificial lighting, follow these top tips:

- Make sure your child has at least twenty minutes outside in natural daylight every day. Research has found that for babies in particular, being exposed to natural light in the early afternoon leads to significantly better sleep at night.[16]

- Try to avoid artificial light sources (particularly energy-saving LED bulbs), and, once the sun sets and it begins to get dark, keep lighting as dim as possible in rooms your child is in in the evening.

- If possible, keep the nursery or sleep room light-free; if this is not possible, use a red light source.

- Keep the last two hours before bedtime 'screen free', with no television, computer games or the like.

- Daytime naps should be taken in a light room, with the curtains open and blinds up.

Scent

The evocative properties of scent are well known. Think how the smell of freshly mown grass can make you feel happy, how lavender can make you feel calm and how citrus smells can make you feel more alert. How about the memories brought back by smelling the perfume your grandmother used to wear or the smell of something your mother used to bake when you were a child?

Smell is the sense most closely linked with memory, and we can use this to our advantage when it comes to sleep. The most reassuring smell for a child is the scent of their parents, their mother in particular, especially if she is breastfeeding. This means that if we can replicate our scent in close proximity to our child they may feel more comforted. There are other ways to use scent to improve sleep, too: see my top tips below.

- Wear an old T-shirt for several nights in a row (at least three or four) and then allow your child to take it to bed with them to cuddle, or use it as a pillow case. For babies, you could cut up a smaller piece so as to avoid any suffocation hazards.

- If your child has a comfort object, keep it close to your skin for several days to allow your scent to transfer to it: try not to wash it. If you do, you will have to re-condition it (see page 112).

- Use lavender oil in your child's night-time bath. Research has shown that children spend more time in deep sleep after a bath with lavender oil added.[17] Not only that, but the cortisol (stress hormone) levels of both mother and child after a night-time lavender oil bath have also been shown to be significantly decreased. Note: do not use the artificially scented, mass-produced lavender baby bubble baths found in high-street shops and supermarkets. Look instead for a good specialist aromatherapy product that is safe for your child's age (see page 281 for a list of recommended products).

- Use lavender oil, diluted in a carrier oil, or purchase a specially formulated massage oil, for a nightly massage, as part of your child's bedtime routine. Research has found that lavender has a calming effect on babies, which in turn may help them to sleep more easily.[18]

- Place a couple of drops of lavender oil in an aromatherapy fan in your child's sleep space every night. Research has found that lavender has a positive effect on night-time sleep.[19] Again, make this part of your bedtime routine, turning the fan on at the very start of the routine so that the room is scented by the time your child goes to bed. Leave the fan on until you go to bed yourself, to allow the fan time to really scent the room. The constant humming noise of the fan also tends to help children to sleep.

Sound

For many babies and young children, sleeping in complete silence *contributes* to sleep problems. Babies like the reassurance of white noise, the sound of their mother's heartbeat, and they naturally find their parents' voices soothing. Right from the very moment a baby is born they turn towards their mother and father, and, even in a room full of people, they seem to know where we are. I think it is such a shame that we seem to believe that night-time should be as quiet as possible, as we are missing a great trick for encouraging sleep. Here are my top tips for using sound to encourage sleep:

- Sing a lullaby to your baby each night. It doesn't matter what the song is, whether you remember the words, or whether you can hold a tune, your baby won't mind!

- For toddlers and pre-schoolers, make up a bedtime song together and make this 'your' song. The sillier and more unique to your family the better. Sing this song every night to signal to your child that bedtime is coming, and to reinforce the predictability and reassurance of their routine.

- For younger babies, under six months, gentle white noise can soothe them to sleep. There are lots of special white noise CDs on the market, created exactly for this purpose. Leave the CD playing softly on repeat all night, so that when your baby finishes a sleep cycle it will help them to begin a new one. Too often we turn CD and MP3 players off after our child is asleep, thinking that they have done their job – they have, but only for the first sleep cycle. Remember, your child has up to ten sleep cycles per night.

- For older babies and young children, consider using a special alpha music CD. Alpha music is simply music recorded to resting pulse rate (approximately sixty beats per minute) and has been recorded with the intention of relaxing the brainwaves into what is known as an 'alpha state' of relaxation. (See page 281 for suitable music choices.) Music has been shown to have a sedative effect on newborns to five-year-olds[20] and has also been shown to significantly improve the sleep of children.[21] Again, as with babies and white noise, it is important that you leave the music playing all night. After all, you want to help your child to sleep well all night rather than simply for their first sleep cycle.

I think creating a bedtime routine that is as multi-sensory as possible is one of the keys to a calmer night's sleep. However, none of the strategies outlined above, especially in isolation, are magic bullets. Don't expect a piece of music or a scent to get your child sleeping through the night in a few days or even weeks. Using multi-sensory sleep triggers takes time – at least a month to six weeks, to have an effect – and they must be used consistently.

A note on my BEDTIME solution

Many parents, desperate for a quick fix for their sleep deprivation, try the techniques in this chapter for a few days or a week before abandoning them, claiming that they don't work. They won't work in a week or two; you need to use them all for *at least* a month, often longer, in order to condition your child. You also need to make sure that you use them every night.

Gentle parenting approaches to sleep take time to work; if they didn't, it would be clear that we are forcing the child to behave in a way that is unnatural to them. Our goal is to work *with* our children, not against them, and because of this we need to invest a little more time and energy than others would with traditional, behavioural sleep-training methods. Remember, we do not want to turn our child into the 'loser', as desperate as we are to sleep more. We also want any results to be long-lasting, to have a positive effect for years to come, and for this reason we must expect our initial time investment to be greater, too.

You don't need to use all of my BEDTIME solutions; pick and choose which ones work best for you and your family. I believe that 'Expectations' and 'Me-time' are the most vital points to grasp, however, and are essential for everybody.

I have devoted the remainder of this book to the specific sleep issues common to children at various ages. It includes what is normal for a child as they develop and how to gently apply my BEDTIME solution to the unique issues experienced at each stage of development. I have also included some real-life examples from parents who have asked me to help them with their child's sleep. Although my suggestions are unique to them, and are unlikely to apply wholly to you, I hope that they will bring my suggestions to life and help you to decide which to apply to your own family.

Chapter 7

Sleep from birth to three months

I could probably summarise this whole chapter by stating: 'Don't expect much sleep!' When I was pregnant with my first baby I truly believed that all newborns did was cry and eat and sleep very little. I was pleasantly surprised then when my son was born that I did get some sleep and there were several hours every day that he didn't cry. I think it's safe to say early parenting exceeded my expectations, though I know it isn't like that for many people whose expectations are more optimistic than mine.

If you think about the changes a baby goes through in their first three months of life 'earth side', it's hardly surprising that their sleep is so erratic! They have gone from being inside the womb, borrowing the circadian rhythm of their mother, enclosed always in the safety and security of her womb, to being on their own, without the hormonal regulators of sleep. The missing circadian rhythms and lack of close physical contact with their mother is not the only thing that has changed though: here's a quick summary of the differences of the womb world and the world as we know it.

A BABY'S ENVIRONMENT PRE- AND POST-BIRTH

In utero	After birth
Constantly held by the mother. Never alone	Estimates suggest babies spend only 40 per cent of their time in physical contact with their parents
In warm water	In cold air
Curled in a foetal position	Laid flat on their back
Almost constant movement	A large proportion of the day spent still
Never hungry, all nutritional demands met via the umbilical cord	Thirst and hunger experienced for the first time and, in many cases, it is necessary to cry to have these needs fulfilled
Very dark	At least half of the day is very bright
Naked	Clothed
Hears mother's heartbeat, blood flow and digestive noises constantly	Lots of different noises, many loud, or complete silence in contrast, especially at night
Sleep/wake cycle shared with mother	No concept of night and day
Impaired ability to smell	Many different smells, some strong, most new

We know that it takes at least twelve weeks for a newborn's circadian rhythms to mature enough for them to be able to distinguish night from day. This is a normal developmental milestone that cannot be hurried so there is little we can do but accept that newborns will wake regularly. We also know that newborns have a very short sleep cycle and experience more REM sleep than any other age group, which means that when they are sleeping they are liable to wake easily.

We can, however, use what we know about a baby's in-utero experience to help us replicate this environment, in order to help them sleep for a little longer and to stay calmer in between sleeps. This concept is known as the 'fourth trimester'. If pregnancy is divided into three trimesters, each lasting for three months, then the first three months of life form another trimester, one in which the baby makes a huge transition between worlds. Simply put, if we treat a newborn baby as if they were still in our womb then life becomes a lot easier and a lot calmer for all.

SUGGESTED SLEEP ENVIRONMENT FOR A NEWBORN TO THREE-MONTH-OLD

At this age the sleeping environment is all about replicating the womb and keeping the baby safe. Therefore my suggestions for a good sleep environment at this age are as follows:

- Keep stimulation to a minimum, so no mobiles over cots or toys on cot bars.

- Follow the SIDS guidelines on page 17.

- At this age, babies should not have a pillow or cot bumpers.

- Put baby to sleep in a sleeping bag or swaddle wrap (see page 128) with no loose blankets in the cot.

- Keep lighting to a minimum at night and rooms naturally lit in the daytime to help establish circadian rhythms.

- Try playing some gentle white noise, such as a CD on low volume throughout the night.

- Consider using a good baby sling or carrier for baby's naps.

The fourth trimester – the key to better sleep with a newborn

How can we replicate the world the baby experienced in the womb? The key is to take each of the differences in their environment before and after birth and try to recreate the same environment as much as possible.

Recreating an environment of constant physical contact

Imagine how unsettling it must be for a baby who is curled tightly in his mother's womb, every part of his body touching hers, suddenly to be born and within minutes to be placed alone in a set of scales or a crib. Most babies experience this within their first hour of life and from their perspective it's all downhill from there. I have lost track of the amount of times I have heard a new parent say, 'My baby won't ever let me put her down – help, what am I doing wrong?' The simple answer is that you are doing nothing wrong. Babies have come from an environment where every second of their existence has been spent being held by their mother, so of course they are going to protest when we try to put them down. We are so consumed with the guilt and fear of creating a clingy baby, making a rod for our own back and not creating bad habits that we rarely hold babies as much as they need to be held. It is completely impossible to spoil a baby, particularly with too much love and too many cuddles. In fact, the more physical contact and nurturing a baby receives from his parents in the critical first few months of life, the more his brain will grow and mature and the more chance he has of being truly independent when he is older. Quite simply, hugging grows brains.

Replicating a constant holding environment

Understandably, most parents wonder how they can fulfil their baby's needs while also fulfilling their own. As lovely as it is to hold a baby all day, it is pretty difficult to go to the toilet, eat, wash and get dressed. Here you have a few options, from asking for help so that somebody can hold your baby while you do what you need to do, to bedsharing if you both want to get some sleep. Babywearing and swaddling can also help.

Babywearing

When I am asked which one baby product is an essential for all parents, my answer is always a good baby carrier or sling. Look for a carrier or sling that supports your baby's hips in a naturally flexed position; in this position a baby looks a little like a frog, with their knees brought up level with their hips. The illustrations below show the correct 'm' position of the baby's hips and legs, and the 'c' shape you are looking for when the sling is in the final position.

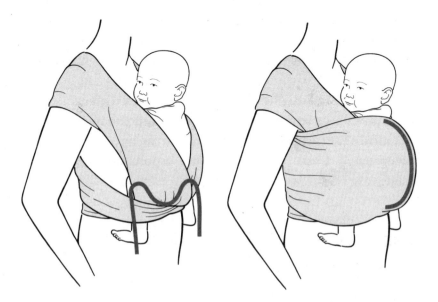

The sling should be supportive for both the baby and for you. At this stage, I recommend using a stretchy wrap sling rather than a more conventional structured baby carrier, as they are softer and hold newborns in a much more natural position (see page 280 for some good slings to look out for). Research has shown that babies who are carried regularly cry significantly less than those who are not.[1] In my experience, they also sleep significantly more and for longer. Perhaps the main benefit of babywearing, however, is having two free hands, enabling you to go to the toilet, eat some food and get on with your normal day ... while your baby is getting all of his needs met.

Swaddling

Wrapping a baby in soft fabric can replicate the womb to some extent and help them to feel more secure. Swaddling is highly controversial at the moment, however, as many believe that it carries risks. This is true – like most things in life, it is not risk-free and if you want to swaddle your baby it is really important that you follow the safety guidelines outlined below. However, if you are mindful of the risks of swaddling and reduce them as much as possible, you and your baby can still benefit from it.

If you are bedsharing and babywearing then the chances are you won't need to swaddle your baby: indeed you should never swaddle a baby who is bedsharing, as this can put them at risk of overheating. If you are not bedsharing, swaddling can be invaluable. It is vital to remember that the goal is not to wrap really tightly from head to foot, in the manner seen in old photographs of tribal cradle boards and the like: modern-day swaddling is much looser, with only a small amount of tightness over the baby's stomach. You're really just trying to create the snug feel of being enveloped in a warm uterus, not trying to create a strait-jacket effect. You can buy many different swaddling blankets and wraps today, most of which have been designed with safety in mind. The illustrations on pages 130–31 show a simple way of swaddling that is mindful of any potential risks to the hips or breathing. The guidelines for safer swaddling are as follows.

GUIDELINES FOR SAFER SWADDLING

- If you are breastfeeding it is important that you do not miss your baby's feeding cues, which may be more likely when they are swaddled. Swaddling can also interfere with the initiation of breastfeeding so do not start until you are confident that breastfeeding is going well.

- Select a swaddle wrap or blanket that is thin and made from natural materials, such as 100 per cent cotton or bamboo fibre.

- Begin swaddling before your baby is ten weeks old. Research shows that swaddling after this may negatively affect a baby's arousability, which could put them at greater risk of SIDS.[2]

- Stop swaddling immediately that your baby can roll; you should only swaddle your baby until they are four months old.

- Make sure that the fabric is not pulled tightly over the baby's chest in such a way that it inhibits their breathing.

- Make sure that the fabric is loose over the baby's hips. They should be able to bring their legs up in their natural frog position easily.

- Never cover your baby's head with the swaddling blanket.

- Do not swaddle your baby if they are ill or have a fever.

EASY 5-STEP SWADDLING TECHNIQUE

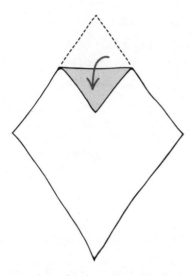

Fold over the top of the swaddle
sheet to make a triangle

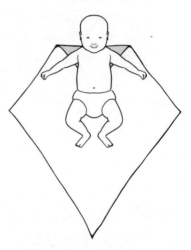

Place your baby with the top of
the fold level with his neck

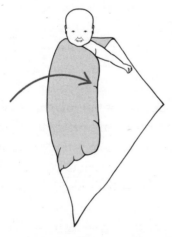

Tuck your baby's right arm at his side,
take hold of the top left-hand corner
and bring it down and over your baby.
Tuck the sheet under his left-hand side

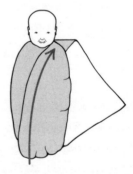

Bring the bottom of the sheet up to
the baby's left-hand shoulder, hold
the baby's arm to his side and tuck
the fabric underneath his arm,
torso and bottom

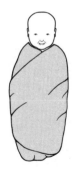

Now, bring the last remaining flap of material to your left and wrap it all the way around your baby, using his own weight to keep the wrap secure

Ensure the fabric is wrapped loosely over the baby's chest and hips – you are looking for tightness over the arms and tummy only

Replicating a warm aquatic environment

Do deep hot baths relax you, especially before bedtime? If you're a 'bath person' you won't need me to convince you of the relaxing properties of being submerged in warm water. This is the environment a newborn is used to, then all of a sudden they find themselves in cold air. Imagine how strange that must feel. The good news is that it is fairly easy to replicate this environment by giving your baby a deep bath in warm water (around 37°C). I find the easiest way of doing this is to get into the main bath with your baby, as this also has the added benefit of physical touch. Sharing a bath with your baby enables them to relax in a foetal position, rather than the rather unnatural position of laying them supported, stretched out on their backs in a conventional baby bath. When my babies were tiny, either myself or my husband would bathe with them every evening (without any product added, to preserve their delicate new skin) as part of their bedtime routine. I also resorted to 'emergency baths' on several occasions – when I knew my babies were overtired but they weren't calm enough to sleep – and it worked like magic.

Replicating the curled foetal position

Have you ever noticed how a newborn will lie naturally with their legs pulled up and their arms pulled in? Many mistake this for the baby being in pain, but in most cases this position is the normal way for new babies to lie when they have yet to uncurl. When you hold your baby tummy to tummy on your chest you'll notice they naturally bring up their legs and adopt this position, just as they do when you carry them in a wrap sling. Imagine how strange it must be for babies to be put down to sleep flat on their backs. There is no denying that placing babies on their back is vital for reducing SIDS risks, however, it's obvious they don't like it very much.

There are two ways to get around this, one of which I have already mentioned, namely carrying your baby on your chest in a sling for naps. The second is sharing a bed with your baby or using a co-sleeper crib at night. In both cases, this allows the baby to adopt a much more natural foetal position. If you are not babywearing or bedsharing it is absolutely essential that you put your baby to sleep on their back and that you are never tempted to put them on their stomach to sleep. SIDS research has found a huge correlation between sleeping a baby prone (on their stomach) and cot death,[3] which researchers attribute to a restriction in the baby's airway and a reduction of swallowing when they sleep on their stomachs.[4]

Replicating the constant movement in the womb

Have you ever lain in a hammock and been lulled to sleep by the gentle swaying? This is what it must feel like for a baby inside the womb. Imagine the gentle rocking the baby experiences when the mother walks. It must be like spending most of your life cocooned inside a blissful, swaying hammock. After they are born, however, we try to keep babies as still as possible, fearful that they may develop bad habits if the rocking that comes to us so instinctively continues. The fact is, rocking a baby is one of the best ways to lull them to sleep, so too is dancing and going for a brisk walk. There is no harm in any of these, whatever others may say. Just because a young baby needs the security of the movement he felt in the womb, it does not mean he will form bad habits if you give it to him. In time, as he grows, his brain will mature and his time in the womb will become more distant and he will need the reassurance less.

If your arms are tired from all of the rocking or you wish there was another way to help your baby to sleep, try dancing around the house with the baby in a sling, or take them outside for a brisk walk. Some parents like to use battery operated swings and others use hammocks for their baby's naps.

One trick I have learned is to make sure that you don't immediately stop rocking, dancing or walking as soon as you think your baby is asleep. At this stage they are probably in a light sleep state and may wake easily when they realise that they are now still; so continuing to gently rock, walk or dance for ten more minutes will ensure that they stay asleep after you put them down or stop moving.

Replicating the constant feeding in the womb

In the womb, your baby didn't know what it meant to be hungry or thirsty, so these feelings are entirely new to him. Everything a baby needs is provided on tap (or rather 'on umbilical cord') in the womb. They have never needed to cry to indicate their distress at having an empty stomach. Imagine how hard it must be to be born and to suddenly experience these unpleasant feelings.

Moreover, think how horrible it must be for a baby whose parents are 'trying to stretch out feeds', even by just five or ten minutes. That's five or ten minutes of the baby trying to tell you 'I need help, my tummy feels funny' and you not responding. Whether you are breastfeeding or formula-feeding, it is so important that you are led by your baby's demands for food.

I don't like the phrase 'demand feeding'. I think it adds to the bizarre notion that babies are manipulative and fighting for control by demanding food, now! It is much better to think of it as 'cue feeding', which reflects the fact that parents are watching their baby for their hunger cues so that they know when to feed them.

Many sleep experts advocate setting a feeding routine early on, in order to get a baby sleeping through the night by four months. This is just not realistic. It does not stop the baby from feeling hungry or uncomfortable, it simply makes them give up trying to communicate their needs. Feeding a baby on demand does usually mean more awakenings than a baby fed to a schedule, but research shows that those fed on demand cry significantly less than those who are not,[5] which I think is a very worthwhile trade-off.

Replicating the constant darkness of the womb

I think this one is pretty obvious. What is perhaps less obvious is your baby's perspective on the world. Imagine lying in a Moses basket looking up at the ceiling and being unable to look away from the bright electric light directly overhead. Or lying in a buggy looking up at the bright sun, unable to shield your eyes. What about a camera flash pointed in your face? If we think of a baby's perspective on the world, we suddenly see how light can adversely affect them in ways we might not have imagined. In the evenings, when the sun sets, we should honour that natural darkness wherever possible, especially in the room where we want our baby to sleep.

Replicating the nakedness experienced in the womb

How strange it must feel for a baby, who is used to nothing more than warm water touching his skin, to suddenly be wearing a scratchy nappy or have a press stud against his skin. How odd it must feel to wear socks or shoes and a hat. I don't know if what a baby wears impacts on their sleep, but common sense tells me that if they are uncomfortable it's quite possible that it does. For this reason I prefer to dress my babies only in soft cotton sleep suits, particularly for the first twelve weeks, when they are transitioning to the feel of wearing clothing. If a baby is comfortable in soft natural fabric, without any restrictions such as waistbands, collars or the like, it must be easier for them to sleep.

Replicating the constant noise heard in the womb

The sound of waves crashing on a beach is one of the most wonderful things about going on holiday. The same sort of sound also calms young babies, reminding them of their mother's heartbeat and the whooshes and flowing noises her body makes from the inside. There are many ways of reassuring babies via sound, from holding them close to our chests where they can hear our heartbeat, to using specially composed 'white noise' CDs and apps to soothe them. Remember that this noise needs to be present for as long as you would like the baby to sleep for, in order to be effective. The noise should be present when the baby wakes between sleep cycles, almost as if you are saying 'It's OK, I'm still here, you're safe to go back to sleep'.

Replicating the lack of smell in the womb

In utero, surrounded by water, it is natural to assume that a baby cannot smell. Once they are born, however, they encounter smells for the first time. In utero, they taste: they practise swallowing amniotic fluid and the smell of this same fluid has been shown to have a calming effect on them. Research has shown that babies who are exposed to their amniotic fluid after birth cry significantly less than those who are not, with scientists concluding that 'the foetus may become familiar with chemical cues present in the intrauterine environment'.[6] It is said that amniotic fluid has a faintly sweet taste, similar to that of breast milk. It follows that, to babies, the smell of their mother, and especially her milk, will be especially calming. It's not surprising then that they show a strong preference for their mother's scent.[7] One obvious way to help calm a baby to sleep therefore is to hold him skin-to-skin to the mother's chest, enabling him to not only feel her warmth and hear her heartbeat, but also to smell her.

A NOTE ABOUT DUMMIES

Many parents ask me if they should offer their newborn a dummy and whether there are any drawbacks if they do use one. This is an area in parenting where there really is no cut-and-dried answer. For many babies, particularly those who are bottle-fed, a dummy can dramatically calm them and help them to sleep, while others may not take to one and, for some, particularly those who are breastfed, the risks certainly outweigh the benefits.

Pros of dummy use

- Can help to calm a fractious baby.

- Can help a baby to begin a new sleep cycle.

- Limited research shows dummy usage may reduce SIDS, but it is commonly critiqued by professionals who question its validity, especially the fact that the research was sponsored by a dummy manufacturer.

- Can give parents of bottle-fed babies a good way to calm their baby if the baby only wants to suck rather than feed.

Cons of dummy use

- Can inhibit the establishment of breastfeeding.

- Can cause orthodontic problems.

- Can cause ear infections.

- Can become addictive – and hard to get rid of – and cause sleep problems once the baby is older.

If you decide you would like to use a dummy with your baby here are my suggestions for how to do so:

- Wait until breastfeeding is well established. Don't use a dummy for the first month if you are breastfeeding.

- Only give your baby a dummy when they really need it (for instance, if they are crying) and take it away as soon as your baby is calm, to prevent dummy use becoming habitual.

- Try to get rid of the dummy by the time your baby is six months old. Any longer than this and it's likely to be tricky to wean your baby off it.

- Some babies really don't take to dummies. If your baby is one of them, don't persevere with trying to get them to take it.

What to expect of your baby's sleep from birth to three months

Nobody really knows how much sleep a newborn needs and, at best, the guidelines are estimates based on educated guesswork and do not account for individual differences.

What to expect at birth

After birth, babies take what is known as a 'recovery sleep', meaning that they can often sleep for several hours, which frequently lulls new parents into a false sense of security. In the first few weeks, babies sleep an awful lot, both day and night. In the first month, babies spend around 80 per cent of their day asleep.[8] Most newborns get between sixteen and seventeen hours' sleep in any given twenty-four-hour period.

What to expect at one month

At the age of one month, babies take an average of three to four naps per day, totalling around seven hours.[9] Total twenty-four-hour sleep is around fifteen to sixteen hours, which is divided between 45 per cent in the daytime and 55 per cent at night.[10] At one month, most babies wake between three and four times a night.[11]

What to expect at two months

At two months, total sleep per twenty-four-hour period averages around fifteen hours.[12] Daytime sleep is around five hours, with around nine to ten hours taken at night, meaning that daytime sleep has now reduced to 35 per cent of the total sleep taken in a twenty-four-hour period, with 65 per cent of sleep happening at night.[13]

What to expect at three months

Research indicates that, by the age of three months, 58 per cent of babies are capable of sleeping for stretches of up to five hours. However, this means that 42 per cent are still not sleeping for longer than four hours straight.[14] Other research indicates that 46 per cent of all three-month-olds still wake regularly every night.[15] Daytime naps begin to decrease in frequency and length at this age, although just over 10 per cent of three-month-olds do not take daytime naps every day.[16] Average sleep per twenty-four-hour period is now around fourteen hours, with around 75 per cent of this now taking place at night,[17] indicating the development of a circadian rhythm.

Making sure feeding is going well

Of particular relevance in the first three months is how feeding is going, particularly if you are breastfeeding. Many sleep problems have their roots in feeding difficulties, the main culprits being a bad latch, and tongue and lip tie. In all cases it is likely that feeding will be painful and the baby unsettled, both on the breast and off. They are likely to be hungry and find it difficult to settle, and their sleep is likely to be adversely affected, both day and night. It is particularly important that you consult a lactation consultant if you are breastfeeding, to check that there is nothing wrong with your latch and that your baby doesn't have a tongue or lip tie, causing feeding difficulties. Tongue tie can affect babies who are formula-fed and, in such cases, a visit to a lactation consultant is important.

WHAT IS TONGUE TIE?

Tongue tie occurs when the baby's tongue is held too tightly to the base of their mouth. This occurs because the frenulum, the piece of skin connecting the tongue and mouth, is too short. Often babies with tongue tie will have a heart-shaped tongue and may find it hard to poke their tongue out; however, the tie can also be posterior, or at the back of the mouth, which is harder to spot.

The lasting effects of the birth experience

One possible effect on infant sleep that is not considered nearly enough, by parents or professionals, is the impact of the birth itself. Birth can have very real and lasting physical and psychological implications for the baby and the mother, and the well-being of each can, understandably, affect the other, especially when it comes to sleep.

Babies can often suffer from lasting physical effects from their birth if it has been via caesarean section or was an assisted delivery, such as ventouse or forceps, as well as when the labour has been either especially long or the baby has malpresented (is lying in a difficult position, or stuck). The impact of their head being constantly pushed down into a pelvis at an awkward angle for the duration of the labour can leave babies in quite some discomfort. They can also suffer from torticollis (severe stiff neck) and are left unable to turn their head. Aside from the discomfort caused, this can also have an effect on feeding, meaning that a baby will not feed from one breast or cannot move their head in such a way as to get a good latch. In addition, they may sleep with their head to one side only, which can put them at risk of plagiocephaly (flat-head syndrome). Understandably, this discomfort can have a detrimental effect on sleep.

Cranial osteopaths and chiropractors also talk about the movement of the baby's cranial bones during labour. As the baby's head moulds, to enable him to fit through the birth canal, the cranial bones move and overlap. The bones usually return to their normal position over a period of a few days following the birth, mostly via the process of the baby sucking, which moves their upper and lower jaw, and this in turn stimulates the base of their skull via their palate. Sometimes,

142 · The Gentle Sleep Book

however, things don't return to normal and an abnormal skull compression becomes noticeable as a result of the baby's feeding habits and need to suck much more than usual. If the baby's vagus nerve (the cranial nerve directly linked to digestion) is compressed this can also have noticeable effects on a baby's digestive system, causing pain. All of this is more likely to happen if the labour is long, the baby is malpresented or is born via emergency c-section, forceps or ventouse. For babies who have had a difficult birth and are fractious, a visit to a good chiropractor or cranial osteopath can make a profound difference, especially to the baby's sleep.

Birth doesn't just affect the baby, of course; it also affects the mother, often profoundly. So many facets of the pregnancy and birth experience can be perceived to be traumatic, indeed the birth doesn't have to be 'traumatic' or dramatic in order for it to negatively affect the mother. It seems that the greatest impact on the mother's perception of her birth experience is not the actual mode of birth itself; it is how she was treated during the whole experience. The most important factor is the amount of control she felt during the birth. Birth can be a scary, lonely and undignified experience and whatever others say about the birth, how the mother feels can be quite different, and rightly so. Experiencing a traumatic birth can impact profoundly on the experience of parenting. As we know already, babies pick up on their mother's stress and a baby's distress affects the mother, leading to a vicious circle of stress and anxiety. I often find that babies who sleep particularly fractiously have had a traumatic birth in some way and the mother has some unresolved trauma.

I cannot emphasise enough how important it is for parents to look after themselves. Too many parents sacrifice their own emotional well-being in a quest to look after their baby, but this self-neglect can often make the early days much harder for everyone. It is paramount that if you have any residual trauma from the birth you talk about it with someone (see Resources, page 279 for details). It might seem bizarre to suggest that talking about your birth experience will help your baby's sleep to improve, but the link is there and in my opinion it is a very strong one.

A NOTE ON COLIC

Colic is said to affect around 20 per cent of all babies. It peaks at around six weeks of age and rapidly subsides by twelve weeks. Often babies seem to suffer more in the evenings between the hours of 5pm and 10pm, with many constantly crying and being incredibly difficult to settle. The official definition of colic, according to the Wessel criteria (named after the doctor who invented it), is a baby that 'cries for more than three hours a day, for more than three days a week, for over three weeks'. This definition is commonly used in medical circles for diagnosing infantile colic, but it is important to note that colic is not a disease or even a medically recognised disorder. It is simply a label given to unhappy babies, where the cause of their crying is unknown. In essence, therefore, there is no such thing as colic.

This is something I strongly agree with. I am not saying that there aren't babies between six and twelve weeks who are very unhappy and cry an awful lot. There are. But I do not believe that there is one cause, nor do I believe that they are crying because of some mysterious gastrointestinal problem or pain. I believe that colic, as we know it, is a label given to far too many babies who are suffering with many different problems, such as:

- tongue tie

- breastfeeding latch problems and oversupply issues

- cow's milk protein allergy or lactose intolerance

- cranial compression or neck pain from the birth

- difficulty adjusting to life outside of the uterus, particularly the lack of holding and separation from their parents

- parental anxiety and stress

- overstimulation and overtiredness.

To cope with colic I suggest following the fourth trimester 'womb to world' points earlier in this chapter (see pages 125–36), coupled with a visit to a lactation consultant or breastfeeding counsellor. Colic is incredibly common and not something you have caused. Perhaps the most important thing to remind yourself is that it will not last for long!

Birth to three month case studies

Here are a couple of case studies from parents I have worked with. I hope these examples help to bring some of the ideas in this chapter to life. Do bear in mind that the answers I have given to these parents and their families may not be appropriate for you and your child, but you should still find the advice helpful.

Julie and Harry, twelve weeks

Dear Sarah,

I would be very grateful for some advice regarding my son's sleep. My little boy is twelve weeks old and has an older brother who is two. Harry was born by emergency caesarean due to concerns about my scar from my previous section and Harry's heart rate. I didn't labour but was having regular tightening. Harry was delivered at thrity-seven weeks and five days in poor condition requiring resuscitation at birth (initial apgar 3).

I breastfed for two days but eventually turned to formula as I found breastfeeding too painful. This had also been the case with his brother. My concern with Harry is that he is showing very similar sleep traits to his older brother. He is very difficult to settle at night – night-time is his most wakeful time of the day. If he is swaddled he seems easier to settle but this is becoming problematic with increasing age as he is now able to free himself from the blankets and I have concerns about the safety of this as I have found him with the blankets over his face on a couple of occasions. He currently sleeps in either a sleep sac, I would like to say in his cot, but in reality he spends much of the night in our bed! I would like to try a routine with Harry but in all honesty his brother's night-time behaviour means that we are more focused on trying to get him to settle.

I am exhausted by both Harry and his brother's night-time antics, which at the moment is like a tag team . . . one settles and the other wakes. I feel emotionally drained by it all and spend most of my day tearful and stressed. Any advice would be gratefully appreciated.

Many thanks

Julie

My BEDTIME solution

Working through my BEDTIME solution, I came up with the following plan for Julie and Harry.

Bedsharing/co-sleeping: Julie mentions that Harry won't sleep alone in his cot, but he will sleep in her bed. As Julie is formula feeding, it is not recommended that she share a bed with Harry due to an increased SIDS risk. Consequently, I asked Julie if it was possible to arrange Harry's cot to be a co-sleeper. I felt this would work really well for the family, as it would give them their bed back, but provide Harry with the close proximity to his parents that he needs.

Expectations: I wanted to make sure that Julie knew what was normal for a child of Harry's age; that at his age it is very normal for a baby to wake regularly at night. Night-time is naturally the time of day that babies are most fractious, particularly a small baby like Harry, and because his circadian rhythms are still very immature and only just beginning to form properly, day and night are very similar to him. After the end of a busy day (and even a quiet day at home will be busy with a toddler around), babies often end up over stimulated and find it hard to switch off. Another tactic I discussed was spotting Harry's early tired signs and trying to get him to drift off. I suggested that if Julie could catch the tiredness before Harry becomes desperate then he will likely become much easier to settle. I also suggested that Julie could consider carrying Harry in a sling in the evenings, 'wearing him down' to sleep while also attending to her toddler's needs.

I was interested in developing Julie's idea of a schedule, in terms of a bedtime routine and helping Harry to know that bedtime was approaching, particularly with a lively toddler around. I pointed out that because Harry was so young it would take him a while to cotton on. I suggested they start with a warm bath each night (just water, no bath products, to prevent his skin from becoming dry), followed by ten minutes of massage and then feed, cuddle and change into a different babygro. I stressed that this wouldn't work miracles, but over time it would begin to make a difference.

Diet: Given the painful breastfeeding, I wondered if Harry had a tongue tie, especially as Julie had difficulty breastfeeding her first son – and the condition can be hereditary. In addition to this I asked Julie to check for any intolerance of cow's milk protein, which would not have disappeared after the switch to formula milk. I also made sure that Julie knew that cluster feeding (feeding regularly in the evenings) was normal for a baby of Harry's age, and not a 'problem' to solve.

Transitional object: I suggested that Julie try to condition the use of a comfort object with Harry – keeping it in close contact during feeds and cuddles, and sleeping with it for a few nights to build up her scent – to help him feel a little more secure.

IT/screen time: It's worth considering whether Harry is exposed to too much television, given he has an older brother. The exposure to the light it emits could impact on his evenings.

Me-time: What struck me here was Julie's birth story. I wondered how this had been affecting her and if it was having an impact on her emotional state, which Harry could be picking up on. Also, it is feasible that Harry may have some head compression as a result of his birth, so I asked Julie to consider cranial osteopathy or chiropractic treatment for him.

I also asked what support Julie had in the form of close friends and family. Two small children is a lot to handle on your own and it struck me that Julie would benefit from some extra help so that she could rest and nurture her own needs, as well as those of her children. I knew her parents were already helping out, but I felt she would benefit from much more regular help, if possible, on a daily basis. The most important advice I gave to Julie was 'start with yourself'. She needed to treat herself kindly and to 'debrief' her birth by talking it through with somebody trained to listen. I also asked if there was any possibility of hiring in some help or, if that was not possible, if she would consider asking for help from a volunteer organisation such as Homestart (see Resources, page 279).

Environment: I asked Julie to be really mindful of the environment that Harry slept in and to consider the use of different sleep triggers, including:

- making sure she and Harry got outside, in natural light, for twenty minutes every day around lunchtime
- carrying Harry in a sling for his daytime naps, to help him to feel secure and to block out some of the external 'noise' (this would also allow Julie to have two free hands to take care of her toddler)
- stopping swaddling, as Harry, at twelve weeks, was approaching the limit with regard to safety
- any daytime naps in Harry's cot should be taken with the curtains open in order to help set his body clock
- in the evenings, artificial light sources should be limited as much as possible, with no artificial light in the bedroom at night (or, if Julie really felt the need, to use a red bulb)
- trying a white noise CD in the bedroom during Harry's bedtime massage and feed; to be left on at a low volume all night
- using lavender oil in an aromatherapy fan in the bedroom as part of Harry's bedtime routine, leaving it on until Julie went to bed.

Update

A few weeks after giving Julie my suggestions I received a message from her saying that Harry's sleep was now better. Harry had since seen a consultant who had diagnosed him with lactose intolerance and advised Julie to change his diet to a dairy-free one. It is likely that this had been affecting his comfort and therefore his sleep. Hopefully Harry's sleep will continue to naturally improve as his circadian rhythms and sleep cycles mature.

Emma and Jacob, ten weeks

Dear Sarah,

I am a first-time mum to Jacob who is ten weeks old. I am loving being a mum but am struggling with helping Jacob to sleep. He sleeps for a maximum of three hours in a block at night-time and only cat naps the rest of the time, often waking minutes after I settle him down.

I do not have a set routine in place for Jacob as I prefer to be guided by his needs at this young age. I do however try to follow the same pattern every evening at bedtime, to help him begin to recognise the transition from day to night. I take him to bed at approximately 9pm, speak to him in a soft, soothing voice, dim the lights and use white noise in the background. I currently lightly swaddle him and have him lying next to me in bed. I am very aware that the swaddling will soon have to cease as he learns to roll. I feed him and then lay him down when he is dozing off (not fully asleep) but this can take two or three attempts. He frequently stirs and becomes upset once laid down, to the point where I need to pick him up to soothe him and/or feed again. The bedtime process can take up to two hours. Once eventually asleep he will stay that way for up to three hours, more often than not waking at 2.30am. When he wakes I try not to rouse him too much, feed him and attempt to resettle him. This process can take an hour. Again he appears to wake himself up within minutes of laying him down and at this point rarely goes back to sleep properly. He may doze for a few minutes at a time but grunts, wriggles around and wakes frequently. If I lay him on my front he will drop back to sleep but I am nervous of then falling asleep myself and also of creating 'bad habits'.

During the day he will often fall asleep at the breast after a feed. However, if I try to transfer him to his hammock or another area for a nap, again he wakes within moments of being laid down. I try to soothe or resettle him but he becomes increasingly agitated to the point where he is wide awake again. He will occasionally calm if I put him in a sling but then requires me to keep moving! It is very normal for him to nap only if we are out in the car or if I let him sleep on me following a feed, where he will happily stay for up to two hours.

Jacob was born via emergency c-section. This was not the gentle birth I had planned! Having started to labour it was discovered that he was undiagnosed breech and he was born via emergency caesarean section weighing 9lb 2oz! I was grateful for his safe arrival but unprepared for how to cope physically and emotionally following a c-section delivery. We live in a rural area, and while my husband and parents have supported me, I have found the isolation hard. I have only just started to get out and about independently.

Prior to his arrival I knew I wanted to breastfeed. When he was born he latched on immediately. The early days of feeding were hard going. He is a hungry baby and at that time I doubted my body's ability to keep up with his demands. Sometimes even now it feels as though I am unable to satisfy his hunger, especially when he thrashes around, head-banging and pulling at my breast. I have recently had mastitis, which made feeding incredibly painful, but I was determined not to give up and have continued through it.

Another factor that has been a challenge is that Jacob was born with a tongue tie. The midwives, health visitor and lactation consultant all told us he would not be treated as he was feeding well and gaining weight. However, I became increasingly concerned that he was presenting with symptoms of reflux and that he was agitated when feeding and his sleep pattern was becoming more troublesome. I eventually had to request a referral to the consultant and have had the procedure to resolve the tie done privately. Since having the procedure a week ago there are signs that his latch and feeding are improving, but there is no change in his sleep as yet.

He is a healthy, alert boy who is beginning to interact with us in lots of fun ways and is starting to take a real interest in his environment – smiling and chatting with us. I try to get out for walks or to visit family each day. My husband works twelve-hour days, six days a week, so I provide the majority of care for Jacob.

I am concerned that he is not getting enough sleep, particularly at night and that it could have a detrimental effect on his development. I am also worried that I am seemingly unable to settle him for naps or after he wakes for his night feed. If I were to let him sleep on me following a feed I know he would sleep for more hours! It feels as though his sleep pattern is getting worse rather than better. I am just about coping with the sleep deprivation but would love to see a light at the end of this tunnel. I want to enjoy every aspect of being Jacob's mum but feel that his sleep trouble casts a shadow at times.

Emma

My BEDTIME solution

Working through my BEDTIME solution, I came up with the following tips for Emma and Jacob.

Bedsharing/co-sleeping: I asked Emma if she would consider proper bedsharing, following safety guidelines, both for naps and in the evenings. I pointed out that she was right to not let Jacob fall asleep on her chest: this isn't safe as he could roll off Emma, or she could fall asleep. I suggested that the side-lying 'cradle' position (see page 98 for a diagram) adopted by breastfeeding, bedsharing mums may well suit Jacob.

Expectations: I reassured Emma that Jacob's sleep was perfectly normal for his age and suggested that we tend to have high expectations of a small baby's sleep because of what we hear from other parents, professionals and the media, especially as a first-time parent. The reality is that a young baby has pretty unreliable sleep, sleeping for short periods of time at a stretch and waking frequently. Emma can be reassured that this behaviour is normal (and healthy) and Jacob's sleep patterns are in line with what you would expect from a ten-week-old.

I also pointed out that night-time is naturally the time of day that babies are most fractious. Jacob is small and as yet his circadian rhythms are still very immature and only just beginning to form, so day and night are very similar to him. I discussed the fact that after a busy day adjusting to 'being earth side', Jacob may be a little over stimulated and find it hard to switch off. Little babies naturally also want as much physical contact with us as possible and that, to Jacob, his mother makes him feel secure, therefore without her warmth, smell and hold, he's naturally unhappy and less relaxed.

I also suggested Emma might try wearing Jacob in a sling for naps, and when putting him down that she wait until he enters a deeper stage of sleep, approximately 20 minutes after he has fallen asleep. I asked Emma to watch out for Jacob's body relaxing and becoming heavy and possibly his eyes moving. Usually in this stage of sleep, babies don't wake up when you put them down.

I suggested that now would be a good time for Emma to begin to implement a bedtime routine for Jacob, consisting of a bath, massage, feed and cuddle. Although Jacob is very young and unlikely to respond much to this yet, it would get them into a really good routine for the future.

Diet: In relation to Jacob's corrected tongue tie, I pointed out that it takes time for there to be a noticeable effect on sleep, but now that feeding was a little more settled hopefully that would help. I also stressed that cluster feeding is totally normal and not a sign of an inadequate milk supply, as some mothers perceive it to be. Emma is doing a great job!

Transitional object: I suggested that Emma might like to try to condition the use of a comfort object with Jacob, keeping it in close contact during feeds and cuddles and sleeping with it for a few nights to build up her scent. This may help Jacob to feel a little more secure, but Emma should remember that he is still very young and adjusting to the fourth trimester, and right now what he really needs is his mum.

IT/screen time: This is not particularly relevant to Emma and Jacob as he's so young and there are no older siblings around.

Me-time: I was struck by Emma's birth story and suggested she might like to talk through Jacob's birth with somebody when she is ready. I felt it could help, particularly given the dramatic change of plan. I also suggested Emma could consider cranial osteopathy or chiropractic treatment for Jacob, given his c-section delivery.

Given her husband's long working hours and the amount of time Emma spends alone as Jacob's sole carer, I wondered if Emma had any support from family or friends. I also asked if there was any possibility she could hire in some help, or if that was not possible if she would consider asking for help from a volunteer organisation.

Environment: I asked Emma to consider the use of different sleep triggers, including the following:

- making sure she got outside, in natural light, with Jacob for twenty minutes every day around lunchtime
- any daytime naps in Jacob's cot or hammock should be taken with the curtains open in order to help set his body clock
- in the evenings, I suggested Emma limit artificial light sources as much as possible, with no artificial light in the bedroom at night (or if she really felt the need, to use a red bulb)
- playing a white-noise CD in her bedroom during Jacob's bedtime massage and feed, and leaving it on a low volume all night
- using lavender oil in an aromatherapy fan in the bedroom as part of Jacob's bedtime routine, leaving it on until she went to bed herself.

A couple of months after sending Emma my thoughts, I received the following update from her.

Emma's update

I am very grateful for the advice you sent me. It was great to receive some practical ideas that fell in line with my natural instincts. I was fed up of people telling me to try controlled crying or top up with formula (they still tell me that!). Your advice has been incredibly beneficial. We now have a vague pattern in the evening, really just so Jacob recognises that it's bedtime. He has a bath at 8pm, then a massage followed by a quiet, final cuddly feed with just a night light on. He does tend to drop off at the breast but transfers easily into his hammock and stays asleep. We have introduced using white noise overnight, which seems to help him stay settled.

Chapter 8

Sleep at age three to six months

You've survived the fourth trimester and your little frog-legged newborn is really showing her personality and rewarding you with smiles and laughs. This period can be a magical time, when your baby is so much more fun to be around. On the sleep front, her circadian rhythms have kicked in and she probably has some sort of discernible pattern to her sleeping and eating. Your baby may now be sleeping for stretches of four or five hours during the night, if you are lucky. The days of cluster feeding and colic are almost all in the past and you are finally beginning to feel confident in your parenting abilities. You may be regaining some semblance of normality in your life and feeling a bit more in control than you did in the early weeks.

Mother Nature, however, has a funny way of making sure that we don't become too complacent with our parenting. Just when you think things are on the up and 'sleeping through the night' may not be such a distant dream, your baby turns four months old and everything begins to deteriorate. You notice that your baby is beginning to sleep like a newborn again, perhaps worse. On top of that your baby can be grouchy and unsettled, but when you pick her up to soothe her it doesn't seem to have the magical effect it did in the early weeks. All of a sudden you begin to doubt your parenting abilities, just as you dared to think you were doing a good job. What on earth went wrong? Or, more precisely, what did you do wrong?

Perhaps your baby is teething? Her clothes are constantly wet and covered in dribble. She also puts everything into her mouth. Or perhaps she needs weaning; perhaps that's why everything is going into her mouth, perhaps milk alone isn't enough any more and the constant night waking is because of hunger? If you're breastfeeding you may be beginning to doubt if you have enough milk.

Getting back to normal is a double-edged sword, too. While it's nice to regain some semblance of a routine, the early days of becoming a new parent are quite special, with all of the congratulations and visits. Now you don't have a newborn any more you may feel you're no longer considered, or treated, as if you or your baby are special. People no longer coo over your baby at the shops; the midwives and health visitors have stopped visiting. The congratulations cards have long since been taken down, the presents have stopped and the visitors have ceased to come. The latter may be a blessing in disguise, of course, since all your relatives have no doubt been asking how your baby is sleeping, before giving you their particular solution. It appears that parents of four- and five-month-olds are expected to know what they are doing and get on with it, without the help that was offered in the early months.

What to expect of your baby's sleep at three to six months

An average three-month-old still wakes 2.7 times each night, and this increases slightly to waking on average 3.1 times each night by the time they are six months old.[1] By the time they reach six months old, babies sleep for an average of fourteen hours in any twenty-four-hour period. The average four- to six-month-old goes to bed at 8pm and has three hours of daytime naps,[2] giving them a ratio of around a quarter of their total sleep taken during the daytime and three-quarters taken at night.

Research looking at the sleep of six-month-olds found that only 16 per cent regularly sleep through the night, meaning that 84 per cent do not. Further research found that by three months of age, although 71 per cent of babies have slept through the night at least once, many relapse into more frequent waking after they turn four months old.[3] In addition to this, 16 per cent of six-month-olds have no regular sleeping pattern at all.[4] In short, between three to six months of age it is normal for babies to wake lots at night. In fact, it is more normal for them *not* to sleep through the night than it is for them to sleep through, which is shocking considering how many endorse sleep training from twelve weeks of age.

Why do three- to six-month-olds sleep so poorly, given that they now have a functioning circadian rhythm? Here are some of the commonly espoused reasons, some myth, some real.

Teething

Most babies cut their first tooth between six and ten months of age. While most parents tend to report that their babies suffer from pain and sleep disturbance during teething, this is not actually backed by research.[5] Often parents mistakenly think teething is the cause of their baby's sleep and behavioural changes.

Most babies begin to really dribble between three and four months old. Many attribute this to teething, but it is actually due to their new-found developmental obsession with putting everything in their mouths, and the maturation of their salivary glands. Babies are hard-wired to explore objects with their mouths, from their hands to toys, which is rarely related to teething. Dribble also contains digestive enzymes and due to the rapid development of the baby's salivary glands at four months of age, this is secreted more prolifically, indicating a baby's growing potential to digest solids within the next few months.

Weaning

How many times has somebody told you that your milk isn't enough to satisfy your baby, or how you need to give them more than just formula milk? We seem obsessed with filling babies up in order to get them to sleep through the night. This is naïve on so many levels, from the mistaken belief that babies only wake due to hunger (they don't), to believing that weaning onto a few spoonfuls of rice or vegetables will provide a baby with more nutrients than milk (it doesn't).

The World Health Organization suggests that babies are ready to be weaned onto solid foods at around six months old. In the UK, the NHS website says that 'Research shows that babies need nothing but breast milk or infant formula for the first six months of life.' A baby's digestive system is not mature enough to cope with anything but milk until they are around six months old and early weaning carries numerous risks. Even after a baby is weaned onto solids, their nutritional needs should be met mostly by milk, which remains an important part of their diet. The early days of weaning are all about introducing taste and texture to babies, not about the amount of food they consume. Some even find that a baby's sleep regresses after the introduction of solids, commonly due to constipation and other digestive discomfort experienced by the baby.

Many people mistakenly believe that when a baby wakes more at night, especially if they take extra milk feeds, they are showing signs of needing to be weaned, but experts agree that this is a normal developmental milestone and not a sign of readiness for weaning at all. The same is true for babies who put everything in their mouths, as discussed above.

True signs of a readiness to wean include:

- being around six months of age

- the ability to sit upright

- the ability to pick up food themselves with their hands and put the food in their mouth

- loss of the tongue thrust reflex, and being able to swallow food. Younger babies who are not ready to be weaned will push everything back out of their mouth with their tongue.

Developmental spurts

This is the real reason why three- to six-month-old babies tend to sleep so erratically. Developmentally, so much is happening at this age. Just think about all of the new skills your baby now has and how quickly they have developed them. This is a time of enormous change and development, not just the obvious physical growth, but, more importantly perhaps, in the brain.

I vividly remember what it is like to parent four- and five-month-old babies. This age was perhaps the hardest with all four of my children; not just because of the broken night-time sleep, but during the day, too. Although I felt sorry for myself, because of the sleep deprivation and frustration I felt while trying to calm my babies, I realised that I felt far more sorry for my babies. At four or five months, babies are much more alert and they seem to understand so much more, but their bodies are still effectively pretty useless: they can't sit unaided, can't crawl and can't stand.

Although they can now pick objects up, they won't be able to let them go again for a couple of months. Can you imagine how frustrating that must be? It may be hard parenting a four- or five-month-old, but imagine how hard it is to *be* a four- or five-month-old!

So much happens developmentally between the ages of three and six months. Physical strength develops rapidly and babies become much stronger and more able to do things, such as grasp and move their body with purpose. Their vision continues to improve and, with it, their hand–eye coordination. Sensory processing matures dramatically at this stage too, which is why everything gets put into their mouths, perhaps the most sensory area of the body because it is capable of touch and taste.

As they near the end of their first six months of life, babies become much more aware of their surroundings. With this new awareness comes the ability to recognise people. Do you remember when your baby was a newborn and would happily be cuddled by anybody? Now they want you, and only you, because they recognise you and, perhaps more importantly, they realise when you are not holding them. Further leaps in brain development kick-start language acquisition, with the emergence of babbling at around this age. All this happens in just twelve short weeks, so imagine how exhausting and confusing that must be for your baby. It's like you learning to speak Russian, acquiring a black belt in karate and becoming fluent in sign language in only three months: pretty amazing and a bit mind-blowing all at once!

As well as being amazing, this dramatic development can also be quite scary and unsettling for babies, leading them to need your presence and comfort perhaps a little more than they needed you previously. I imagine it's a bit like you've emigrated to somewhere with an entirely different climate, a different language and different food. You would probably feel pretty unsettled, not to mention confused. How might you react to such an upheaval? Would it be fair to say that you might want to cling to those you love or those things that remind you of home? Would it be fair to say that you might be a little cranky in your new overwhelming world of change? Would it be fair to expect that due to all of this upheaval you may find it a little hard to sleep? With all of the new experiences running through your mind it would be pretty hard to switch off, especially when you do finally get to sleep and then wake up in strange surroundings only two hours later. Perhaps you might crave the comforts of home as reassurance? To your baby you are their home; indeed you were their home for nine months, so it's only natural that they want to be with you more.

I think this is how life is for a three- to six-month-old, especially when things come to a head at four to five months, the peak developmental-spurt age. Try to imagine how overwhelmed your baby is feeling. In many ways, as exhausting as it is, he is giving you the ultimate compliment by telling you that he needs you, and you are the one thing in the world that helps him to feel safe and secure. Can you imagine though, amidst this upheaval, introducing solid foods? Moving a baby into their own room or starting sleep training? These things would surely add to your baby's stress. I strongly believe that the key to surviving the four- to five-month developmental spurt is to change as little as possible.

In fact, if anything needs changing at this stage, it may be in the way you treat yourself. This stage will pass, but you must be kind to yourself, as well as your baby, while you are going through it. What support do you have? Can you ask anyone to help you? What might you be able to put on hold for the next few months while you help your baby navigate this critical period of their development? It is vital that you take care of yourself now and keep reminding yourself that this stage *will* pass.

SUGGESTED SLEEP ENVIRONMENT FOR A THREE- TO SIX-MONTH OLD

At this age, the sleeping environment is about a gradual move away from womb-like surroundings to an environment where the baby is becoming more comfortable with short separations from its parents. My suggestions for a good sleep environment at this age are as follows:

- Keep stimulation to a minimum at the earlier end of this age range: no mobiles over cots or toys on cot bars. Older babies may enjoy something that makes their sleep environment more fun, but still try to keep stimulation to a minimum.

- Continue to follow SIDS guidelines (see page 17).

- At this age, babies should still not have a pillow or cot bumpers.

- Put the baby to sleep in a sleeping bag with no loose blankets in the cot. Swaddling should stop before the baby is four months old.

- Keep lighting to a minimum at night and rooms naturally lit in the daytime, to help establish circadian rhythms.

- Babies may still benefit from some gentle white noise, but at the older end of the age range they may benefit more from relaxing music left on softly all evening or nap time.

- This is a good age to introduce a comforter if the baby does not already have one, tied to the cot bars in order that it does not pose a hazard to the baby.

- Consider naps in a good, supportive baby carrier.

- If your baby has one, try to wean them off of their dummy by the end of this period.

A note on crying it out and crying in arms

For many parents this can be a really difficult time, particularly when their best efforts to soothe their baby fail. Many worry that they can no longer soothe their baby's cries and wonder what they have done wrong and why their previous fail-safe methods no longer work. I have come to the conclusion that sometimes babies need to cry and sometimes, as parents, the best thing we can do is to be with them and to allow them to cry while we are there for them.

I do not mean that you should leave a baby to cry alone in their cot, or in a different room, even if you are periodically returning to check on them: this is something I do not agree with. What I mean is that sometimes babies seem to need to cry and we need to accept this and not worry about stopping the crying all of the time. So long as you are calm and your baby is in your arms, held lovingly, I believe that allowing them to cry is fine. In fact, sometimes it is better than fine because occasionally babies simply seem to need to release their frustrations through their tears. Effectively, when you hold them and allow them to cry, what you are saying is 'It's OK, I hear you, I'm here for you, you're safe and you are loved, I can be strong enough for you to express your emotions.' Many parents, particularly dads, feel that they have somehow failed if they are unable to stop their baby's tears, but sometimes I think being able to just 'be' with a crying baby is helpful to them, and definitely not a failure.

Three to six month case studies

Rosie and Arthur, four months

Dear Sarah,

My four-month-old son, Arthur, has been sleeping in our bed since day one and I'm worried that he will find the transition to sleeping on his own hard if we don't start taking steps soon. How do I move him from our cosy bed to his cot without tears – from either of us?

He still feeds frequently – every two to three hours, but less during the nights when my partner is not sharing the bed with us. I'm concerned that Arthur may be waking up more frequently at night than he needs to due to our co-sleeping – too hot or too cramped! When me and Arthur have the bed to ourselves he only wakes up once or twice. When his dad is with us, it's more like five or six times. I love co-sleeping but fear it is stopping Arthur from getting a good night's sleep.

He is exclusively breastfed and he took to it easily. We battled with ductal and oral thrush for almost two weeks, which made feeding very painful but co-sleeping meant I at least felt rested. In fact, my night feeds were less painful, perhaps because I was lying down and relaxed.

His birth wasn't easy. I had planned a hypnobirth and all was going to plan. I was 4cm dilated and in the birthing pool at my local midwife-led unit. Four hours later, I hadn't progressed at all and was strapped to a trolley and put in an ambulance to the nearest consultant-led unit in the next town. I was scared and lost control of my pain at this point and asked to have an epidural ready on arrival. They agreed and gave me an epidural and put me on a syntocin drip to speed up my contractions. I fell asleep but was woken up minutes later to be told baby's heart rate had dropped and they were setting up the theatre just in case. The obstetrician examined me and despite only being 8cm, she started guiding Arthur out and I started pushing. Long story short – he was very big – 10lb 6oz – and got stuck at his shoulders. When he came out he had the cord round his neck and wasn't breathing. They quickly resuscitated him on the other side of the room. All I wanted was to have him with me but, as I had torn badly (3rd degree) and was losing blood, they took me to theatre, leaving Arthur with his dad!

An hour after he was born, I finally met my baby and got the skin to skin I knew we both needed. He latched on quickly and I didn't let the midwife dress him for another four hours! As I'd had the epidural, I couldn't get up and put him down myself, so I just kept him with me. He was very sleepy and didn't suckle much, but I was pretty out of it so was happy for us to snooze together. That night, he slept on my chest in the hospital and I just stared at him! When we got home, I didn't want him out of my sight. We arrived home in the evening and when it came time to put him in his Moses basket, it felt wrong, so I took him to bed with me. He has been with us ever since.

After a few weeks, my partner started suggesting we start putting Arthur in his Moses basket to get used to it. He was way too big for it already, which I was secretly pleased about. I was also pleased that he woke frequently for feeds in the night. He lost ten per cent of his birth weight by day three and never got back up to his line on the WHO centile graph, but I always knew he was getting enough milk.

Our routine and average night:

7am wake up, feed in bed

7.30am up, chat and sing songs, get dressed

9am nap – either walking to a group or feed to sleep in bed

9.30am baby group or play time

BF whenever asked for during the day

11/12ish nap – either on boob or in pram

Afternoon unstructured, but usually a nap on the boob or fed to sleep in bed if he seems grouchy and tired at some point

6.30pm stories, bath, massage, zipped into sleeping bag and then:

7pm white noise on mobile (cot is right next to bed) turned on. Breastfeed in bed

7.30pm asleep

8.30pm occasionally wakes up and falls asleep as soon as I start feeding him

10pm I go to bed. This always wakes him, so I feed him back to sleep

12 occasionally wakes up – feed to sleep

1am always wakes up – feeds

3am usually wakes up – feeds to sleep

5am always wakes up – change nappy and feed to sleep

If he is still awake when he finishes a feed, I can rock him to sleep on the bed by putting one arm under his legs. If I unlatch him when he's sleepy, he wakes up unless I rock him in this way.

At four months, Arthur is hitting all the milestones he should. He's very smiley and chatty, is good at picking things up and holds big soft things between his thumb and forefinger. He can't roll, but wriggles a lot and I often find him at funny angles in the bed.

I don't really want him to leave our bed but I worry that co-sleeping is benefiting me more than him. Also, I wonder if the nature of his birth has made me worry too much about not having him within arm's reach. He seems like an outgoing, happy little chap and I don't want my insecurities to tarnish that.

I hope you can help me with strategies to make the move away from co-sleeping as tear-free as possible! I still like the option of having him in with me if my partner is working a night shift (a fortnightly occurrence) or if teething/illness means Arthur is feeding more. I hope you can help!

Thanks for reading,

Rosie

My BEDTIME solution

Here are my thoughts for Rosie and Arthur, based on my BEDTIME solutions.

Bedsharing/co-sleeping: I began by asking Rosie how she really felt about sharing a bed with Arthur, and whether her concerns were more to do with societal expectations and the opinions of others, or if she really did want to move him out. She replied that she loved sleeping close to him and would like him to stay exactly where he is. My advice was that she didn't have a problem. If she was happy, and her partner too, then it doesn't matter what anybody else thinks. Worrying about the future only makes the present less enjoyable and needlessly difficult. Baby Arthur has only been in this world for four months, and there is plenty of time for him to sleep alone in the future. At this age, close contact with parents enables babies to become truly independent at a later stage. They will often move into their own sleep space of their own accord, where their sleep will often be much better than that of their contemporaries who were moved away from their parents before they were ready.

I helped Rosie to understand that babies who bedshare with their parents (and breastfeed) sleep 'normally'; that is their sleep is lighter than those who sleep alone and are formula-fed, and to compare the two is unrealistic. The trouble is trying to combine the demands of modern-day life with a primitive infant and their primal needs.

I suggested that if Rosie's partner found it difficult to sleep with Arthur in the bed that he may consider sleeping in a different bed for a couple of months until Arthur's sleep naturally improved, or that they could consider using a co-sleeper crib if they wanted their bed back to themselves.

Expectations: Arthur's sleep is normal for a baby his age. I explained to Rosie that we tend to expect a lot more of babies' sleep because of what we hear from other parents, professionals and the media. The reality is that a young baby has unreliable sleep; they sleep for short periods of time at a stretch, wake frequently and feed regularly throughout the night. All of this is normal and healthy. Any guidelines about how much sleep a baby should have are entirely that, guidelines – there is no science behind them, just guesswork!

I explained that as Arthur matures he will naturally need Rosie less. As his circadian rhythms and sleep cycles mature, his sleep will lengthen and become more reliable naturally, but these are all developmental stages and for that reason cannot be rushed.

I also pointed out that the age of four months is a notoriously tricky time for sleep. With all of the developmental changes happening for a baby, it is very normal for their sleep to regress at this age, but that the good news is that he won't always be like this and things will get easier naturally.

With regard to Arthur's routine, I commented that this was a great idea and Rosie's routine seems very natural and sensible, but to remember that Arthur is still very young and it is going to take him a while to cotton on. Therefore Rosie should not be disheartened if the routine doesn't have a magical effect. She should be consistent and do things in the same order every day which, in time, Arthur will pick up on and take reassurance from. The real advantage of routines is that they set things up well for the future.

I suggested that Rosie should look out for Arthur's early tired signs, both for daytime naps and in the evening, and should work with these as much as possible. Preventing Arthur from getting overtired will help him to go to sleep more easily and, importantly, he may stay asleep for longer.

Lastly, I suggested that if Rosie was happy to rock Arthur to sleep then not to worry about changing anything for the time being. Similarly, if Arthur falls asleep on the breast, Rosie has a great tool for getting him to sleep. In the future, when Arthur is approaching about twelve months old, she may want to move towards helping him fall asleep without the rocking or the breast but, for now, if she's happy, she should just keep doing what she's doing.

Diet: It seems that breastfeeding is going smoothly now, after the initial hiccup with thrush. Arthur is still a couple of months off of weaning age so I didn't feel this category was especially applicable to Rosie.

Transitional objects: I suggested that Rosie may want to try to condition the use of a comfort object, such as a blanket, muslin or cuddly toy, so that Arthur has good associations with an object for the future, should Rosie need to leave him or want to put him down without nursing him to sleep when he is older.

IT/technology: I don't think this is particularly applicable to Rosie and Arthur, but I suggested that she try to avoid having him around TVs and laptop screens from 6pm, in order to not inhibit his night-time sleep.

Me-time: I was interested in Rosie's birth story and her thoughts about it. Science has proven that babies pick up on their mother's emotional states and I wondered if Rosie's experience has affected her emotionally. If so, it may be that Arthur is picking up on this and is fussier and harder to settle as a result. My suggestion to Rosie was to treat herself kindly; to have a birth debrief if she needs to, by talking through it with somebody trained to listen (see the organisations listed on page 279); and to nurture herself as much as she nurtures Arthur. Rosie needs to eat well, sleep and rest whenever she gets the chance. I asked if she might consider hiring in help if it was financially viable. If that was not an option, I suggested that she might ask for and accept help from family and friends or contact a charitable organisation that could provide free help for young families (see page 279). In relation to Arthur's birth, I asked Rosie if she had considered cranial osteopathy or chiropractic treatment for him, in case he was experiencing any lasting physical effects.

Environment: For daytime naps, I asked Rosie if she had considered carrying Arthur in a sling, which would give Arthur the contact that he needs while allowing her to use her arms. Or it might be possible for Rosie to join him for a daytime nap in bed, which would allow her to catch up on sleep herself.

I suggested that Rosie should try to get outside with Arthur, in natural light, for twenty minutes every day around lunchtime.

Daytime naps should be taken with Arthur in natural light (curtains and blinds open). I mentioned that in the evenings Rosie should try to limit artificial light sources as much as possible, with preferably no light at all in the room that Arthur sleeps in. If Rosie does use a light in her bedroom she should make it red-based. Also, I suggested that in the lead up to bedtime Rosie should limit the lighting in the rooms that she and Arthur are in as much as possible, using dimmer light switches and lamps. I also suggested that Rosie may like to try playing white noise softly all night, not turning it off when Arthur falls asleep, which will help him to return to sleep when he wakes between sleep cycles.

I received the following note from Rosie a short while after sending her my suggestions:

Rosie's update

Dear Sarah,

That was the answer I was hoping for. I love sharing a bed with Arthur and on nights like last night where he was waking up a lot to feed because he has a cold, I couldn't imagine having to keep getting up. My other half seems to think he'll sleep through if we put him in his cot but I think the opposite will happen!

I'm going to carry on trusting my instinct and move him when it feels right. It really doesn't yet and I would only be doing it because of pressure from other people. Another thing I hadn't thought about – Arthur's dad has mild sleep apnoea. I have no idea if it is hereditary but I know that co-sleeping can only be a good thing if it is.

He will move into his own bed one day, but we're all very happy co-sleeping now. Thank you so much for your help.

Hannah and William, five months

Dear Sarah,

I have a twenty-week-old baby boy, William, who has woken frequently in the night from birth. Me and my partner are exhausted as we also have an energetic two-year-old who needs our attention.

Our son arrived after a very fast and very 'easy' labour and birth. I was in very slow early labour for about four days. I had fairly regular but not particularly painful contractions so I was able to carry on as normal. I went to bed on the fourth night and within the hour I was woken up having very strong contractions, so we made the journey to the birthing centre. I was examined and jumped into the birthing pool, and within minutes our son had arrived. No pain relief, no medical intervention and I was able to enjoy a psychological third stage with plenty of skin-to-skin and a natural start to our breastfeeding journey.

William is exclusively breastfed, with the exception of three bottles of formula one night due to illness at about two weeks old. He was born with a tongue tie, a lip tie and a high palate and we are also currently waiting on the results of some allergy testing as it is possible that he has an intolerance to lactose, soya and eggs. His tongue tie was divided at six days old and his lip tie was divided at about six weeks old, after I suffered severe nipple trauma and often bled. He fed for very long periods of time and frequently, there was one day in particular that he was latched on for a period of about ten hours, screaming during my rushed toilet breaks.

From birth he has struggled to sleep for longer than two hours in one block, often waking somewhere between 30–45 minutes throughout the night, quick 5 minute feed then asleep again. We always would change his nappy to try and wake him up a bit to see if he would feed a little more, hoping that he would sleep a little longer. His feeding during the day improved and now he will happily have a fairly short feed (5–10 minutes) every 2–3 hours but at night his longest stretch would be 2 hours at the start of the night (usually down to sleep between 7–8pm) which then usually becomes every 45 minutes–1 hour until 5.30am. He will feed for about 2 minutes and fall asleep and we will attempt to wake him up by changing his nappy and chatting, turning lights on etc. in the hope he will take a bit more milk but generally he sleeps though this and doesn't take any more.

We currently co-sleep, with him sleeping in a sleeping bag next to me with a bed guard to keep him from rolling off the bed. We do believe that he is teething at the moment but we do not feel that this has had either a positive or negative effect on his sleep pattern so far. We have been advised by our health visitor to start weaning him as this will help with his reflux (possibly caused by his intolerances) but we have yet to take the first step.

So far we have not yet tried much in terms of aiding his sleep; he will happily fall asleep in a sling during the day and so I will carry him for a majority of my day. Neither me nor my partner are comfortable with the idea of sleep training, especially at such a young age, but he is not easily soothed without milk, even though he often doesn't take a full feed. We currently feed him to sleep at night but we don't really have a bedtime routine but often decide that we will 'start one from tomorrow'.

As you can imagine, we are exhausted. I feel comforted knowing that he is seeking me out for comfort during the night but the frequent waking is causing tension as we are all very tired. Our two-year-old often wakes up around 4am and joins us in the family bed which means that we are awake very early because we generally can't sleep when she joins us. William used to be very fussy and would refuse to sleep unless it was on top of me but he seems to have settled somewhat and the majority of the time he seems happy to be laid beside me. I am on a fairly strict diet which has improved his general manner but this hasn't yet extended to his sleeping patterns.

With regards

Hannah

My BEDTIME solution

My suggestions, based on my BEDTIME solution, for Hannah and William, were as follows.

Bedsharing/co-sleeping: Hannah is already sharing a bed with William, which she is happy with.

Expectations: I explained that frequent waking at twenty weeks is very common. I confessed to Hannah that I found four and five months the hardest time in terms of baby sleep with my own children, something that is echoed by many parents around the world. I explained that her son was in the middle of lots of growth and developmental spurts, which usually result in sleep regressions. Due to the issues that she had experienced in his earlier days, Hannah may not have noticed that William's sleep has regressed as it never really improved. William is waking roughly every forty minutes, which is the length of one entire sleep cycle at this age. With this in mind, Hannah needs to look at ways that she can make her son more comfortable and reassured so that he can sometimes begin a new sleep cycle without her help.

Regarding bedtime, I wondered if Hannah was choosing for her son to sleep at 7pm, or if this was something he was doing naturally. If the latter, then great; it's always best to follow a baby's lead when it comes to sleep. If the former, I wondered if it was too early. Babies are put to bed very early in our society and if they are not ready to sleep it can often result in more difficult bedtimes. I understand the desperation of 'needing' a child to go to bed in the evening and having some time to yourself, but often this backfires if they aren't ready for bed. A good natural time would be somewhere around 8pm, which should be enough to make a difference. In addition, a good bedtime ritual is vital. Hannah's son needs time to wind down before bedtime and nap time and to recognise that the time for sleep is approaching. Implementing this as soon as possible and being consistent is very important, so today might just be the day she should finally start!

Diet: It's great that Hannah is investigating whether or not her son has allergies and intolerances. Reflux is a symptom, not the cause, of an unhappy baby and if she can find the underlying cause then she will be going a long way to making both of them happier. I felt it was a great shame that her health visitor only suggested weaning, as often this can aggravate things if the baby is given food to which they are allergic or intolerant. To add to this, under around six months of age, a baby's gut is not mature enough to handle solids and their salivary amylase production insufficient to break down much of it. Hannah may find that she needs to do nothing else if it does turn out to be diet related!

Transitional objects: I suggested that if he doesn't have one already, Hannah could try to condition the use of a comforter, a blanket, cuddly toy, muslin or similar, in order to help William to feel reassured enough to begin a new sleep cycle without always needing her help. To condition the object, Hannah should cuddle it whenever she cuddles William, wear it in her top for a while to transfer her scent and eventually (after a month or so) her son will hopefully associate the object with her.

IT/technology: I suggested to Hannah that she have absolutely no screens on (TV or otherwise) in the house for two hours prior to bedtime. I know this is hard with a toddler around, particularly if you need the toddler entertained in order to see to the baby, but it is so important. Screen time is highly stimulating for babies and children and can inhibit the release of the hormones responsible for sleep, causing disrupted nights.

Me-time: I advised Hannah to do some serious nurturing work on herself. It is very difficult to look after a small child and a baby without either lots of help from friends or relatives, or lots of time seeing to your own needs. I told Hannah that sometimes she needed to put herself first. She might spend one night per week locked in the bathroom, relaxing in a bubble bath with a magazine while her partner babysits, or she could book a monthly massage or beauty treatment or listen to a mindfulness or relaxation CD every day for twenty minutes. I also suggested, if possible, she try to find some physical help, whether in the form of a charity volunteer (see page 279) or a mother's help or postnatal doula if her finances could stretch to it. Whatever she does, I reminded Hannah to bear in mind that it's not selfish to want to recharge your batteries; it's selfless, because it means you're recharging your batteries in order to give more to your children.

I also asked Hannah if she could utilise her partner more on nights when she really needed a good sleep. Perhaps they may consider this just once a week on a Friday or Saturday night, when her partner does not have work the next day. If Hannah feels really desperate for sleep she could move to another room, knowing that her son is in her partner's capable hands, loved and safe. Her partner should respond to his son however he needs to, feeding, holding, rocking, hugging and so on, though he needs to be prepared for the fact that he may cry. Hannah would then concentrate on the important work of catching up on sleep in order that she can care for both her baby and toddler better over the coming days. Given this was likely to upset her baby son, it should be a last resort, when she is at rock bottom, but sometimes it would be necessary.

Environment: I suggested that Hannah should try to make sure she gets outside with her children for around twenty minutes every day, around lunchtime. During daytime naps, Hannah should keep the curtains or blind open in order to build upon her son's natural body clock, in the hope that he will sleep more at night. In the evenings, once it gets dark, Hannah should limit artificial light as much as possible in her home and keep lighting dim, and if she has energy-saving light bulbs she may consider changing them to regular ones in the rooms the children spend their evenings in. She should ideally keep the bedroom free from light, but if this is not possible I suggested she use a red-based bulb only, in order not to inhibit the release of the sleep-inducing hormone in her son.

As William is having trouble beginning a new sleep cycle on his own, I think it is important that Hannah begins to condition some sleep cues, like white noise or alpha music (see page 120) played all night and all nap time (it's important it is played all night, not just at bedtime). I told Hannah that this wouldn't be a miracle cure, and that she must condition it first by playing it when she is feeding, cuddling or bathing her son in order that he associates the music with her presence and feeling calm and safe. I suggested that it would take at least four weeks for this to help.

I also suggested Hannah condition William to a certain scent, in much the same way as she should use music. She might choose to use lavender or Roman chamomile oil in an aromatherapy fan diffuser in the room that her son sleeps in. Again, Hannah will need to condition her son to the scent, by using it in his baths and preferably also for a daily massage. Again, the scent needs to be present for the duration of the sleep. The combination of the music, the scent and a transitional object might help William to feel reassured enough to begin a new sleep cycle without needing her presence every forty minutes.

I received the following update from Hannah a couple of months after giving her my suggestions:

Hannah's update

We now have a great bedtime routine. It's actually helped with our two-year-old, too. It's a really nice time for us all to connect in the evening.

They both settle to sleep really well now. William still goes through times of waking more regularly but he only woke twice last night, which is a massive difference. We have a comforter, but he doesn't seem to have taken to it too well but that's OK. Both kids also have a little dinner with us in the evening. He doesn't eat a lot still but we offer it and I assume he'll start scoffing in his own time. Thank you, you've really helped us.

Chapter 9

Sleep at age six to twelve months

The second half of a baby's first year of life is a lovely time, when their personalities really shine through and the frustration tends to lessen as they gain the skills of sitting upright unaided, crawling, cruising and sometimes walking. I loved introducing my children to solid foods and watching their wonder and amazement as they squished strawberries, chomped on pasta and pulled the funniest faces when they ate something sour or bitter. Many parents have become more confident in their parenting skills by now, and their baby is usually in a natural nap-time routine of sorts during the daytime and, with the baby's circadian rhythm firmly establishing, nights are usually a little easier.

On the other hand, this is commonly the time that maternity leave ends for those who are returning to work and a baby has to cope with the transition to daycare, with whomever and wherever that may be. Combine this with the emergence of the dreaded separation anxiety and parents can often find themselves exhausted and frustrated, wondering if their child will ever sleep through the night and nap reliably in the daytime. This is made ten times worse by the incorrect general assumption that, by the age of six months, babies are capable of self-soothing, should no longer require night feeds and therefore should be sleeping through the night.

What to expect of your baby's sleep at six to nine months

At the start of this period, only 16 per cent of babies are reliably sleeping through the night every night.[1] Around 60 per cent of babies are sleeping for periods of five hours or more with some regularity and 13 per cent still wake at least three times every night.[2] At six months, babies are sleeping on average around 10½ hours at night and 3 hours in the daytime. At this age, babies will be taking around 30 per cent of their sleep during the daytime and 70 per cent at night.

What to expect of your baby's sleep at nine to twelve months

At this stage, babies sleep for around thirteen hours in every twenty-four-hour period: 10½ of these hours are taken at night with 2½ hours composed of daytime naps. Remember that these are just the norms of sleep and some babies will sleep for longer, while some will sleep less. Sleep is split between 80 per cent at night and 20 per cent in the day. This is, however, a very common time for sleep to regress, with night-waking becoming more frequent than it was between six and nine months. Research indicates that now only 40 per cent of babies are sleeping for stretches of five or more hours at night and that the majority are still waking at least once at night and usually needing parental input to get back to sleep.[3]

SUGGESTED SLEEP ENVIRONMENT FOR A SIX- TO TWELVE-MONTH-OLD

At this age the sleeping environment is about helping your baby to feel safe, secure and happy, particularly when they are away from you. My suggestions for a good sleep environment at this age are as follows:

- At this age babies may enjoy mobiles or toys on their cot bars, particularly if they can make them move or do something by themselves. These can be good for entertaining babies when they wake in the morning, which may give you an extra five minutes' sleep.

- It is still important to follow SIDS guidelines (see page 17).

- At this age babies should not have a pillow or cot bumpers.

- Put your baby to sleep in a sleeping bag (babies of this age should not be swaddled), with no loose blankets in the cot.

- Keep lighting to a minimum at night and the room naturally lit in the daytime to help establish circadian rhythms.

- Consider playing some relaxing alpha music (see page 120) for the duration of the nap time or night.

- This is a great age to use a comforter, particularly one that is easy to access and that your baby can cuddle.

- Ideally you will have weaned your baby off their dummy for naps and night-time sleep by now.

- You can still carry your baby in a good supportive carrier for nap times if they need to be close to you. You should look for a supportive structured back carrier (see page 280).

Why does sleep regress at nine months?

It seems so cruel doesn't it? Just as you have recovered from the four- and five-month sleep regression and think you can see light at the end of the tunnel, everything goes pear-shaped again. If you are lucky you might have had several nights of uninterrupted sleep between the six- and nine-month period, but this luxury can spoil you, as it leaves you unprepared for the nasty shock when your baby begins to wake more than they have done for months. To add to this, nap times reduce in length and often in frequency and your baby may not be so happy to be put down for a nap without you any more. Baby sleep often feels like it is two steps forward and one step back, but during this phase it can be more like one step forward and two steps back.

Why is it so common for sleep to be interrupted at this age? The answer usually hinges on two words: 'separation anxiety'.

What is separation anxiety?

Some people would have us believe that this very normal phase of development is the 'fault of the parent'; more specifically, the fault of parents who have made rods for their own backs, mollycoddled and created clingy children. They are wrong. Separation anxiety is an indication that the parents have done a great job. It's a good sign. It shows that the parents have raised a psychologically healthy and completely normal child.

When babies are born, they have no idea that they are a separate entity to their mother. As far as the baby is concerned you may as well be his arm or leg, he sees you as such an integral part of his being. It takes a while for babies to realise that they are separate, but, more importantly, to begin to comprehend that their parents, in particular their mother, can leave them and, potentially, not come back. This knowledge heightens between six and eighteen months, usually peaking somewhere around nine or ten months.

Separation anxiety shows that your baby has formed a secure attachment with you, which is a strong indicator of a normal, healthy personality in later life. In the last century many prominent psychologists spent a long time researching attachment theory. This important work has led them to believe that true independence and confidence in children stem from a secure attachment to their mother (in particular) during their babyhood.

One of the best indicators of 'secure attachment' (the most desirable, and indeed normal, style of attachment) is a baby or young child who is comfortable exploring their surroundings when in the presence of their mother (or father), but who gets very upset when their mother leaves and will only calm when she returns. Society, however, tends to label this child as 'clingy' and sees this as a sign that the parents have not done enough to foster independence: in other words, they have failed their child. This couldn't be further from the truth. Another incorrect assumption made by society is that in order to create a confident, independent child we must encourage them to be independent by leaving them alone for increasing lengths of time. True independence, however, is not learnt through rewards, punishments and sleep training. If you want your baby to be confident and independent, the magic answer is to allow them to form a trusting and secure relationship with you now.

A nine- to twelve-month-old baby whose sleep regresses, who cries for his parents during the night and is reluctant to leave them for a nap during the day is not a cause for concern or an indicator of your inadequate parenting abilities. This behaviour is totally normal and a way of your baby congratulating you on your responsive and empathic parenting. It's a great sign, however exhausting and infuriating it might be.

During this stage it is so important to empathise with your baby and to try to understand that this is a normal phase of development, albeit a scary one, for them to pass through. Keep reminding yourself that your baby is not trying to manipulate you, no matter what anyone else (especially of the older generation) says. Sadly, despite the research into attachment theory in the 1950s and 1960s telling parents that this is a natural and positive step in a child's development, the findings didn't really filter down into mainstream parenting advice. In fact, more babies of that time were probably raised by the advice of Truby King and his contemporaries, which focused heavily on parent-led routines and 'tough love'. Babies were fed strictly by the clock, at three- or four-hour intervals during the day and not at all at night, whether they cried to be fed or not. Babies were put into their own room straight from birth and parents were advised not to cuddle them too much or else they risked spoiling them. Most experts in this era believed that babies needed to be taught to be independent through periods of being left alone. This is the advice that many of our parents very likely grew up with and it is still perpetuated by many today. It's no wonder that so many see 'clingy' nine-, ten- and eleven-month-olds as problematic and a reflection of parenting that has been 'too soft'.

ATTACHMENT THEORY

Many people mistake attachment theory for attachment parenting. Although attachment parenting is based on the psychological attachment theory, it is not the same. Attachment theory hinges on the work of psychologists John Bowlby and Mary Ainsworth, whose work in the 1950s, 60s and 70s explored the importance of the relationship and bond between parent and child.

Mary Ainsworth's famous 'Strange Situation' experiment studied the response of infants to being separated from their mothers and concluded that a child who had a healthy attachment with their mother would show great distress when separated from her and left with a stranger.

One important part of attachment theory is the idea of allowing a child to be attached (not necessarily physically) to their parent when they need to be and then to begin to detach (or what we would call 'independence') when they are ready. A child who is 'attached' to their parent at a young age is more likely to become independent than a child who has independence forced upon them by their parents, perhaps in the form of teaching them to self-settle. This letting go is as important as allowing a child to attach in the beginning, but is misunderstood by so many.

Psychologists have found that the attachment a child has with their caregiver during infancy is a strong predictor of their personality in later life, particularly in regard to the relationships they form with others in adulthood.

How to reduce the impact of separation anxiety

- Consider postponing moving your baby into their own sleep space. Most people are aware that it is safer for babies to sleep in the same bedroom as their parents for the first six months of life. After this, however, many are keen to move their baby into their own bedroom, often in the hope that it will improve their sleep. Keeping your baby in with you for just a few more months can often help your baby to feel more secure, which can actually improve their sleep.

- Consider your return to work. It is very common for mothers to return to work when their child is between six and twelve months. If possible, consider timing your return to work such that your baby is settled in childcare and has formed a close bond with their caregiver before separation anxiety hits, meaning when they are six or seven months old. Alternatively, could you postpone your return until separation anxiety has eased a little, post twelve months? Whenever you return, make sure that your baby has a close bond with their caregiver: for this reason many babies are better with a childminder or nanny than in a nursery environment. If your baby is at nursery, however, it is really important to make sure that they form a strong attachment with their keyworker.

- Help your baby to feel as close to you as possible when you are not there, whether during nap- and night-times or if they are being cared for by somebody else. You can do this through the use of tactile objects, sounds and smells. You could give your baby an item of your clothing to hug, a muslin lightly spritzed with your perfume or even a photograph of yourself for them to look at. You could even record your voice, talking to your baby or singing a lullaby.

- Try to keep the rest of your life as constant as possible during this difficult phase – nine months is not the greatest time to go on holiday, for instance, or to start a trial session at nursery or the gym crèche.

- Be kind on yourself while your baby is experiencing separation anxiety. The real key to surviving this period is you. You can't do much to speed your baby through this stage, nor can you stop them from feeling totally normal feelings, but you can change how you respond. In order to respond with compassion you need to nurture yourself. Sleep when you can; enlist help from people your baby already has a secure attachment with, even if it is just for them to sit cuddling your baby for an hour while you soak in the bath; ask people to prepare meals for you; and consider temporarily employing a cleaner or somebody to do your washing and ironing for you (using our local laundrette's service wash was a godsend for me during this phase with my children). Find something that helps you to mentally relax – yoga, relaxation or mindfulness CDs or downloads, running, reading a good book and long bubble baths are all good.

- Keep reminding yourself that 'this too will pass'. One day in the not so distant future you will look back fondly on the days that your baby needed you so much and smile, I promise.

- The easiest way to survive separation anxiety is with help from family and friends. This was summed up so well by the father of attachment theory, John Bowlby, who said, after his in-depth study of the effects of attachment and separation in the 1950s, 'Just as children are absolutely dependent on their parents for sustenance, so in all but the most primitive communities, are parents, especially their mothers, dependent on a greater society for economic provision. If a community values its children it must cherish their parents.'

Six to nine month case studies

Ellie and Sophia, eight months

Dear Sarah,

I am in real need of some advice about my eight-month-old daughter's sleep at night. She has always been a good sleeper, until a few weeks ago when she developed a habit of waking up at 3–4am unable to soothe herself back to sleep. It started after a bout of teething which obviously interrupted her sleep a lot. So I occasionally started using a dummy from about six weeks and I even almost stopped using it alto-gether. However, her older brother who is six has autism so once this habit started, I would use the dummy at night if she woke so the noise would not wake him.

When she wakes I have tried giving her a cuddle/sssshing her, singing gently, but it just escalates; she does not need milk – although she will always have milk if it's offered and that soothes her. What I do now is give her dummy and she goes back to sleep instantly. If I am lucky it stays in till wake up time at about 6.30am. However, sometimes it falls out and I'm up and down the stairs! I am now at a point where I really need her to sleep through. She has done until recently so it's a dependency on the dummy and a bad sleep habit she has acquired.

I am concerned for my son and not disturbing his sleep, he will become confused and perhaps distressed if he hears her crying for long periods ... I think, it is hard to tell. So that is why the dummy has been useful to a point. I would love to find a way to help her to soothe herself to sleep and eventually get to a point where she does not need or want the dummy. She has a muslin which she nuzzles, which I wish comforted her as much as the dummy. Now we are in a cycle I need to get out of! I am exhausted, so is my husband. We have a very supportive family and a part-time nanny who has been with us six years, but they are not here at 3am. Essentially I need her to sleep well not just for her but for us too. Having a child with special needs is intense and exhausting so sleep is very precious in this house.

A little background on us – Sophia was a planned c-section as my son's birth was incredibly traumatic. The delivery went very well; it was eleven days before her due date. She is a happy, content baby and is formula-fed. I have followed the self-led weaning approach and she loves her food. She naps well in the day (45–60 minutes in the morning, and 1½–2 hours in the afternoon). She is on the cusp of crawling and is developing typically. I am aware of these milestones more than others as my son developed very late and atypically. I follow a routine during the day, not religiously but enough to give her a sense of knowing what her day is like, and she tends to respond really well to it. During the day I use a dummy if she wakes up half way through her nap, so it is only sleep based, never used out of the cot.

Best wishes

Ellie

My BEDTIME solution

After reading Ellie's letter, I thought of the following advice for her and Sophia.

Bedsharing/co-sleeping: I didn't think either bedsharing or co-sleeping was particularly relevant here.

Expectations: Sophia has got into the habit of needing her dummy to comfort her back to sleep when she wakes after a few sleep cycles. While I am all for babies being allowed free access to objects that comfort them, in this case the dummy is the source of both comfort and discomfort, as it is causing Sophia to be distressed when she wakes and it has fallen out. Ellie has a tough choice to make: should she allow her daughter to keep the dummy that comforts her so much but causes issues, or should she wean her daughter off the dummy, removing some comfort initially but helping her daughter to sleep more soundly without it? This is a choice only Ellie can make, which is exactly what I told her.

Sophia's sleep is actually very good for her age. She wakes far less and needs far less intervention from her parents to get to sleep than most babies her age. I thought it was really important that Ellie understood this, as this resetting of expectations can often help parents to cope better.

I also mentioned that Sophia is at a classic age for separation anxiety and it is very common for sleep to regress at this age. Only 40 per cent of babies of Sophia's age are 'sleeping through' the night. This stage is transient and if Ellie's concerns are related to separation anxiety, rather than just dummy habit (which it may well be), it is something her daughter could well grow out of with no intervention.

Diet: I didn't think diet was particularly relevant here, aside from naturally making sure that Sophia wasn't waking due to hunger, which is still very normal at this age.

Transitional objects: In order to wean Sophia off her dummy, Ellie needs to slowly condition her to new comfort objects, such as a cuddly toy or special blanket. This will involve far fewer tears and will be far less stressful for everybody compared to other, more traditional methods of dummy weaning, but it will take a fair amount of time, several weeks, if not months. It is important that Ellie does not take the dummy away until the new comfort object is conditioned adequately. The question here, given Ellie's difficult situation with her older son, is whether the family can cope for this length of time?

IT: I didn't think this was particularly relevant here.

Me-time: Given Ellie's level of exhaustion and the demands of looking after her son I asked if it would be possible for her nanny to work for a couple of nights, or if the family could employ a night nanny or doula for one or two night shifts per week. This would allow Ellie to get a couple of uninterrupted nights.

I also suggested Ellie go to bed very early in the evenings to get a solid chunk of sleep before her daughter wakes. In addition, I raised the importance of Ellie nurturing herself as much as possible.

Environment: Ellie needs to add other conditioned comforters to Sophia's nap- and night-time sleep environment, as these will help to reassure her and provide comfort in place of her dummy. Again, whatever Ellie chooses needs to be conditioned and in place for several weeks before her daughter's dummy is removed. I suggested Ellie use a relaxing music CD, which she should play during bath time, massage, cuddle time and milk-feeding time.

In addition, I suggested Ellie use a comforting scent, such as lavender or chamomile, in the same way in a fan diffuser in Sophia's room and also use the same oil blend in Sophia's bath and for massage. The hope here is that, eventually, she will form a good association with these sleep cues and will not need the dummy. When Ellie finally removes the dummy, I suggested after no sooner than four to six weeks, Sophia shouldn't miss it too much.

My last thought: is Ellie's son around during the daytime? If he is at school, I suggested that Ellie might look at making any changes to her daughter's daytime naps and not her night-time sleep initially. If Ellie could remove her daughter's dummy reliably for her daytime naps, then it is likely to be much easier to remove it in the evening, without tears.

I received the following response from Ellie in relation to Sophia's sleep.

Ellie's update

Wow, thank you very much. Your advice is incredibly reassuring. I really hear what you say about doing it gradually and although I'm knackered it instinctively feels right to do that. That way none of us will experience too much trauma!

I can easily remove the dummy during daytime naps, and knowing that at her age this waking is very common is a relief. I'll definitely incorporate the muslin more and try other comforters during bath/bed routines.

Kirsty and her eight-month-old twin boys

Dear Sarah

I'm really hoping you can help me as I'm just so tired and really need to solve our current sleep problems. I am so tired I snap at my eldest when it's not really his fault which makes me so sad. And I miss him. I want to be able to put the boys down for a nap and then get an undisturbed hour with him to play or read or do craft. Something that's hard to do with his brothers around.

I'm a stay-at-home mum to three children, a little boy aged four and a half and twin boys who are eight months. My older son was a poor sleeper but now sleeps well – he is very much a lark, being ready for bed early and then up early. We sought help with his sleep at nine months old and had support with 'sleep training' but there were lots of tears all round and I don't want to go through that again.

My pregnancy with the twins was quite hard. I was very sick until twenty weeks pregnant and had to take anti-sickness medication and spent a lot of time, often whole days, just resting in bed. Then later in the pregnancy I was very large and uncomfortable and had difficulty sleeping. Because the boys are identical twins there was concern about the placenta's ability to support both babies past thirty-seven weeks so labour was induced at thirty-seven weeks to the day.

The induction took one dose of vaginal pessary and then my waters were broken. From the dose of pessary to delivery of twin one was about fourteen hours. Twin one was head down and twin two was transverse. I delivered both babies vaginally in the operating theatre; we were in there in case twin two needed to be delivered by an emergency c-section. I delivered twin one with the assistance of a midwife and then the registrar turned twin two and I delivered him eight minutes later. No instruments were needed to assist with the birth but I did have a large bleed afterwards and lost over a litre of blood. Twin one weighed 5lb 11 and twin two weighed 5lb 4. After the boys were born we were kept in hospital for a week. I needed two blood transfusions and the boys both lost more than 10 per cent of their body weight and needed light therapy for jaundice. Since then we have all been well and they were seven months old when they caught their first cold.

They have been exclusively breastfed from birth to weaning at six months old. We have taken a more baby-led approach to weaning rather than purée but don't offer only finger foods. For example, I spoon-feed breakfast as I need to get all three children up, fed, dressed and ready to get the eldest to school. Therefore a day's food will be something like banana porridge for breakfast, breastfeed after morning nap, lunch will be something like hummus and toast, selection of vegetables and some fruit or cheese chunks, pitta bread, selection of vegetables and some dates. Dinner could be casserole and they will pick up the chunks themselves, or pasta and sauce which they feed themselves followed by natural yoghurt which I spoon-feed to them. They will breastfeed on demand through the day.

When we came home from hospital we had a bedside cot which the boys shared on my side of the bed. When they outgrew this we took it away and took the mattress off the bed. They now sleep on the double mattress and I have a single one at the side. They have never slept well at night although it did improve from three to four months when they would feed at 11pm and sleep through till 2–3am then feed and sleep again till about 5.30–6am. At four months they began waking frequently and between the two of them I could see every hour through the night. I believed that this was the four-month sleep regression but they never seemed to come out of it!

Our night-time routine at the moment is that dinner is between 5 and 5.30pm. After dinner my husband will bath them and get them dressed for bed. I set up the bedroom with dimmed light and a calming CD playing gently. My husband brings them through one at a time. I start to feed the first one then tandem feed them until sleeping and lay them on the bed. This will be around 7pm. On a good night they will then sleep till about 10pm when I will feed them on waking. Usually they will wake individually so I will lie next to them and feed them back to sleep. From here anything can happen! Rarely they will sleep then till 1 or 2am and then feed back to sleep. By 4am though they will be more unsettled generally and wake more frequently. Often they will not sleep through till 10 and I can be feeding one of them back to sleep anything from 8.30pm onwards. Most nights I will see nearly every hour responding to one or the other. It is good if I get a two-hour undisturbed block of sleep!

Until recently they haven't napped in a cot. The first nap of the day is always in the pram as they are awake from 6.30/7am so by the time we leave for the school run at 8.30 they are tired and fall asleep either on the way there or back. They will sleep in the pram anything from 30–90 minutes. I never wake them unless I have to get them from the pram to the car for some reason. Lunchtime naps have been in rockers or slings but I felt it necessary over the last week to start to move them to a cot for this sleep as it felt unfair at weekends and holidays that my eldest was being told to be quiet downstairs so the babies could sleep. We have built a double cot so they can sleep together. To settle them for the nap in the cot I have tried the following. I take them up to their room. The blind is closed. I put them in their sleeping bags and tandem feed them to sleepy but awake. I then put them in the cot awake, read a short story and sing a lullaby. I then turn on the same music as night-time and shush and pat hoping they will go to sleep. A couple of times I have got them to sleep by putting my head onto the mattress next to them but usually I have to cuddle them and rock them. This process can take an hour or more and they may then only sleep for 20 minutes.

Both boys have their two bottom teeth. They dribble a lot and the top teeth have clearly moved but have not cut through. They wear amber teething necklaces and clearly do suffer at times but we have not had issues like bad nappy rash associated with the teething.

During the day we have a variety of activities. I take them swimming once a week, we go to parent and toddler groups and to a baby signing class. These are all morning activities as by 2.30pm we need to get ready for school pick up. We get home from that by 3.30pm. Often they will feed around this time and then play on the floor while I prepare dinner.

My parents live locally and are still young and well enough to help out. They will attend groups with me, walk them so I can clean the house or get an hour in bed and help in the evenings with the bedtime routine when my husband is away. I find it hard to ask for help after a bad night as I feel they do so much for us already.

Emotionally I feel a bit spent and exhausted. I don't expect them to sleep through but I would love to get a four- to five-hour block of sleep at night and to be able to put them in their cot for a nap with ease. I won't use a cry-it-out method but really struggle with the nap time as, if they both cry, it's hard to comfort them both at the same time. In the night if they wake together I tandem feed them back to sleep. I'd also love them to be settled enough at night so that they only woke once or twice so that either my husband could join us (he's still in the spare room due to the frequency of their waking) or we could move them through to their own room. We tried changing the night-time routine to milk before bath to break the association of sucking to sleep but I cracked on the second night and fed them again to stop the cries!

    Kirsty

My BEDTIME solution

After reading Kirsty's letter I suggested the following for her boys.

Bedsharing/co-sleeping: I was pleased to hear that the twins are sharing a sleep space, after all they spent many months together in the womb and the close proximity to each other now may help to soothe them.

Expectations: I began by helping Kirsty to realise that her boys' sleeping behaviour (both daytime and night-time) is totally normal; that despite what society and the media tell us, eight-month-olds usually wake at least twice every night, need parental help to get back to sleep and often need us just as much for their nap times. Kirsty has already survived the four- to five-month sleep regression. Some babies, however, seem to take forever to come out of this and can be tricky through to seven and eight months of age, then go straight into separation anxiety at nine months. I highlighted that early infancy is a period full of developmental change and growth and that some babies can be extra sensitive to these changes.

    With regard to the twins' days, I asked Kirsty to make sure that they get at least twenty minutes outside every morning. I suggested that she should keep the curtains open for nap time, as the twins need natural light in order to build their natural body clock, so that they will sleep more at night. In the evenings, once it gets dark, Kirsty should limit artificial light as much as possible in the home and keep lighting dim. If she has energy-saving light bulbs I suggested Kirsty might consider changing them to regular ones in the rooms the twins spend their evenings in.

Regarding the twins' bedtime, I wondered if Kirsty was choosing for them to sleep at 7pm, or if they were naturally getting sleepy at this time. If Kirsty chose the time, it may be too early. If babies are not ready to sleep it can result in more difficult bedtimes. I understand the need for a child to go to bed in the evening, to get some time to yourself, but often this backfires if they aren't ready for bed. A natural time for the twins might be between 8 and 8.30pm. I also discussed the importance of a good, consistent bedtime routine.

Diet: I suggested Kirsty might consider giving the boys a small supper half an hour before their bedtime (even after dinner), just in case they were hungry, although, in this case, I think it is unlikely.

Transitional objects: If they don't have one already, I suggested that Kirsty might want to think about conditioning the use of comforters for each twin. She needs to build up an association with whatever objects are used by cuddling the object close while holding or feeding the twins. She could also wear the objects in her clothing for a while to transfer her scent and eventually, in four to six weeks, the twins may associate the objects with her, and gain comfort from it without needing Kirsty.

IT: As Kirsty has a four-year-old, I asked if her television was on much, and suggested that there should be absolutely no TV (or other screen time) for the two hours in the run-up to bedtime. I know this will be hard for her older son, but screen time is highly stimulating for babies and children and can inhibit the release of the hormones responsible for sleep, causing disrupted nights.

Me-time: I asked Kirsty if it was possible for her to get some more support. She sounds like an absolutely wonderful mother, but I just don't think it is possible for her to look after a small child and two babies without considerable help. I know her parents help out already, but I feel Kirsty needs more. She must also put herself first sometimes. This could be in the form of locking herself in the bathroom with a magazine a couple of nights per week; it could be a monthly massage; or listening to a mindfulness or relaxation CD every day for twenty minutes. What she needs most, however, is physical help, whether this is from a charity organisation volunteer, a postnatal doula, a nursery nurse or nanny. At night, this need for help is heightened.

I asked Kirsty if her partner could help more at night. He can hold, rock and cuddle the twins as much as they need on nights when she needs to catch up on sleep, perhaps on a Friday or Saturday night (or both) when he does not have work the next day. This would provide Kirsty with a much-needed break at night. If she is feeling really desperate she could move to another room, knowing her boys are in capable hands, loved and safe. This would allow Kirsty to do the important job of catching up on sleep to enable her to have more energy to care for the twins in the coming days. I think this is the most important part of my advice to Kirsty.

Environment: Kirsty might consider using a red-based night light in the twins' bedroom or, even better, none at all. I also suggested she condition a scent cue, highlighting how important it is to condition it – to help the twins to link it with feelings of calmness and contentment beforehand. Just using a scent without this conditioning is pointless, however relaxing the smell is. I mentioned that this was not a quick process and would take at least four to six weeks of continuous conditioning and usage to make a difference. The same is also true of music. Kirsty must condition strong relaxation links, through the use of massage, cuddling and milk feeds with the music playing, and wait for at least a month of continuous usage and conditioning to see any effect. I also mentioned that the music needs to be playing softly for the duration of the sleep, whether a daytime nap or the whole night.

I received the following from Kirsty a few weeks after giving her my suggestions. I still suspect that the key for this family is in finding some regular support in the daytime and occasionally at night too.

Kirsty's update

Hi Sarah,

They are still not great sleepers but I can see improvements and I've become more accepting of the situation. Most days are OK but I've had a run of being ill and it does feel that with a few good nights' sleep I'd be better.

I stopped trying to get them to nap in the cot. It's basically become a big playpen which they go in if they are awake in the mornings when I need a shower and my husband isn't around. Most of the time they are happy to play in there.

Five days a week we have the school run to do so they always fall asleep on the way there or back. Weekends I still take them out at the same time. After lunch I put them back in the pram and walk again until they sleep. I leave them outside in the pram when I get home until they wake. I would like to be able to put them down in the cot for their naps but I think I've become fearful of the transition. The pram works and they don't cry so it's what I do.

They just have the two naps now, waking anything from 2.30 to 3.30 in the afternoon. With dinner around 5.15–5.30 they have a bath between 6.15 and 6.30ish. At night I still feed to sleep and co-sleep. We still play the CD all night. I use chamomile in the bath and the bedroom. Some nights they settle quickly after their bath, others it can take a long time.

Kirsty

Nine to twelve month case study

Kate and Frankie, twelve months

Hi Sarah,

My son Frankie is twelve months old. He was born healthy at full term and we went home the following day. He is our first child. At birth a tongue tie was diagnosed but he latched on and fed well, although weight loss was 9 per cent and gain slow until the division at two weeks old. During this time I was advised to pump and/or consider formula supplementing, which I decided not to do as I was sure he was supposed to feed little and often and on the occasions he fed really well he would forcibly vomit.

At seven weeks it turned out my instincts were right, he'd been fighting against an obstructed bowel which was now so bad it was cutting off the blood supply and needed immediate surgical correction.

From six weeks to four-and-a-half months, Frankie underwent five hospital stays totalling four weeks. Two major operations and eighteen days of total starvation, i.e. IV fluids only. He was exclusively breastfed until the first op, when, after five days of not being allowed to feed him, I was allowed to feed him my milk via bottle (so they could measure input/output). When finally allowed to breastfeed, Frankie cried and thrashed around. I was scared to push it as he was so fragile after the op, the consultant made me feel quite guilty for not just feeding him by bottle.

I struggled to pump and by this time had hugely swollen, bruised breasts which would only yield an ounce or so after excruciating pumping. Anyway, I continued to attempt breastfeeding once home and eventually Frankie took several feeds a day. Sadly, after so long my supply and his patience was low so four weeks later breastfeeding broke down again.

A few weeks after that we were back in hospital with the same symptoms and Frankie was starved again for a week while they hoped to rest the bowel. This seemed to work and we went home, only to end up in our local A&E the next night with a terrifying night of him vomiting dark green bile and screaming in pain. They frankly messed about trying to do a similar process to the time before until I called the original consultant and arranged an ambulance back to his ward. There they operated the next day and the problems were much worse, and they had to remove some of the bowel.

Frankie recovered for the next week, again no feeding. I tried to keep him asleep most of the time. He had half-hourly observations because of the morphine. We took him home at four-and-a-half-months old, a tiny, weak, floppy little dot. The next month consisted of lots of tummy time and round the clock feeding as he'd lost 1½lbs and obviously hasn't gained any over the past few weeks. He improved rapidly and thank goodness has been healthy since. He is now between 75/91st centile for height and weight, very active and strong and happy.

My only concern is he's never slept more than about five hours but quite frequently four. He often appears to feed (milk) every four hours in twenty-four hours. I often co-sleep with him because I'm trying to cut out night feeds and he is hard to settle without some milk. If I try to give him a smaller amount or water he cries. I have seen improvements from time to time and he used to go down well, although often after a feed. He now will only fall asleep if I lie next to him on our bed. Another point of note is that he often wakes from naps crying uncontrollably. He is also quite sweaty at night, regardless of temperature or clothing.

The weaning process is long and he still gets at least 80 per cent from milk. He is only just 'getting' food and that has reduced milk feeding very slightly. So sorry for the lengthy back story, I just wanted to highlight why I often think conventional methods don't apply and also I'm wary of advice from healthcare professionals, as it has not always been very good! My questions are, is it a sleep disorder? Is it as a result of his hospitalisations or 'starving' or both? And shall I just carry on as I am and hope for the best?

Thanks so much, it felt cathartic to get that down in writing!

Kindest regards

Kate

My BEDTIME solution

The following is a summary of my advice to Kate.

Bedsharing/co-sleeping: Kate mentions that Frankie will only fall asleep if she lies next to him on her bed, but she doesn't mention what happens after this. If Frankie is moved to his own room or his own cot I asked if she would consider sharing a bed with Frankie all night, or at least consider moving his cot next to her bed. While this is very unlikely to reduce the night wakings, as babies who bedshare tend to wake more frequently, it is likely to reduce the stress in the night when Frankie does wake. I reassured Kate that there was no harm in sharing a bed with Frankie and that considering everything he had been through in his short life, Kate too, it may well make Frankie feel more settled.

Expectations: Kate was worried that Frankie had a sleep disorder. I reassured her that I didn't feel this was the case. Frankie is actually sleeping very normally for a baby his age, but societal expectations have led Kate to believe that there is something wrong with him. Frankie is breastfed and we know that breastfed babies generally wake more at night, but it is important to remember that this is the human 'norm' for sleep. I do understand that many families with an older baby reach a certain stage where they feel that they just can't carry on as they are. It would be much easier to be baby-led at night if we didn't have to do anything else or have other responsibilities, but this is unrealistic for most people.

I wondered if Kate had a bedtime routine for Frankie. Implementing a routine now is really important so that Frankie knows what to expect each day. A consistent bedtime routine is very reassuring to children, who like the predictability and structure.

With regard to their daytimes, I suggested Kate make sure that they both get outside every morning. I also wondered how busy their days were and suggested Kate may try scaling back their days a little if she considered them busy. Often I find if parents have a quieter time at home in the daytime, they have much calmer nights.

Diet: I wondered if Frankie may have any food allergies or issues, particularly with relation to his medical history. I therefore suggested Kate speak to Frankie's doctor about any potential links.

I reassured Kate that it was quite normal that Frankie preferred milk to solids at his age; most babies really get the hang of eating solids in their second year of life. I asked if she would consider giving Frankie a small supper half an hour before bedtime (even after dinner) of something like toast or porridge, if Frankie was interested of course.

Frankie's frequent night waking is very strongly linked with his night-time milk feeds. For this reason I asked Kate if she was happy to continue with the night feeds. I think Frankie is still benefiting from these, not just nutritionally, but psychologically too. Night feeding is not just about the milk, it's about the contact and the comfort that this brings. If, however, Kate is desperate to reduce the night feeds and Frankie's subsequent night waking she may want to consider night weaning, in the knowledge that Frankie's sleep is unlikely to change much until he is weaned from the night feeds.

I feel that night weaning should only take place after a baby has turned one, although I do not think there is a set age where all children should be night-weaned. It comes down to how the parents feel: if they are happy to feed in the night until the child is two, three or even older then that is precisely what they should do and should be reassured and supported in their decision. I highlighted to Kate that if she was not yet ready to consider night weaning that the onus would be on her to change her life so that she can better cope with Frankie's night-time needs.

If Kate wanted to night-wean, then my suggestion was to try to calm Freddie at night, before offering the breast. If it is obvious that this isn't going to work, and it usually doesn't, then let Frankie feed, but when he slows and appears to be falling to sleep to take him off the breast. Kate will effectively be giving Frankie the message that he can feed to calm, but not to sleep. Frankie is likely to protest, understandably, so I suggested Kate pick a time when life is pretty quiet. I told Kate that if she does decide to try to night-wean then it is really important that Frankie is not alone, and she should always be with him, offering him comfort. Kate didn't mention if Frankie's father lives with them, but if he does, another option is for Kate to sleep elsewhere for three or four nights while daddy sleeps with Frankie and responds at night. Again, Frankie is unlikely to like this, and is likely to cry, but it is important for her to remember that he is not being left alone to cry; he is safe and loved in his daddy's arms. Parent-led night weaning usually doesn't happen without tears. I suggested to Kate that if reading my suggestions was making her uncomfortable then perhaps she wasn't quite ready to night-wean and she may want to revisit it in a few months.

Transitional objects: If Frankie doesn't have one already, I suggested Kate condition the use of a comforter. Eventually, after at least four to six weeks, Frankie may associate the comforter with Kate, meaning he needs her less at night.

IT: Kate doesn't mention if she has a TV, but if she does I suggested that Frankie has absolutely no TV (or other screen time) for the two hours in the run-up to bedtime due to its stimulating nature.

Me-time: Kate has been through such a lot in the last year with Frankie's health problems. For this reason, and given Frankie's frequent night waking, I strongly suggested she do some serious nurturing work on herself. Kate sounds like a wonderful mother, but it's simply not possible for her to look after Frankie, and go through everything that they have together, unless she looks after herself and, at times, puts herself first.

Environment: I suggested to Kate that in the evenings she limit artificial light as much as possible and keep lighting dim. She might also consider using a light in her bedroom that is red-based or, preferably, nothing at all.

I also suggested Kate should condition some sound and scent sleep cues so that Frankie feels reassured when he wakes after a sleep cycle. This will help him begin a new cycle without Kate's help.

A few weeks after giving Kate my suggestions I received the following from her:

Kate's update

Thanks so much for your fulsome reply, it's so kind of you to take the time. The tips you've listed make good sense, some of them I've thought of but inconsistently and to see them in black and white helps me to see how I could structure the day differently for a start.

I think you're right about the night weaning, I just cannot see a possibility of Frankie being coerced into weaning before he's ready. He settles so well after a feed that it seems senseless to spend hours upsetting us both, time that could be better spent asleep! The only time I think perhaps I ought to be more 'strict' is with regard to his weaning onto solids, that is to say, if he had less milk would he eat more 'proper food' during the day. I'm constantly worrying that he ought to be eating more food and having less milk, he just isn't very into it.

Anyway, I just wanted to let you know that I'm trying a few adjustments to our day to accommodate some of your suggestions, such as the walk out before lunchtime. I'm already trying to pare back our days at the moment to see if it helps with mealtimes. Finally the red light/music is something we've touched on but again haven't done consistently.

I am actually OK with Frankie's sleep at the moment – we can get by now that we co-sleep all of the time. My husband is very supportive too, he just works a lot, but I sometimes wonder if Frankie will ever get a sibling given the current arrangements!

I have wondered about allergy testing as Frankie has occasional odd poos and also a pin-prick rash on his cheeks, forearms and thighs, sort of like dry skin. I will look into it again with the doctor. I will let you know how we get on. Thank you once again for your time.

Kate

Chapter 10

Sleep at age one to two years

Can you remember the days before you had children? When you could go to bed whenever you felt like it, sleep all night and wake late at weekends after an unbroken night's sleep. Doesn't this seem luxurious now? I remember at the height of my parental sleep exhaustion thinking that I would give anything (and I mean literally anything) to be able to get a full night's sleep and a lie-in again. Before I had my children I didn't even begin to think that the disrupted nights and early mornings would persist into the toddler years. Babies wake at night, everybody knows that, but there is an unwritten rule that once they are out of the baby years then everything goes back to normal. Only it doesn't. Health professionals and parenting experts may suggest that if your one-year-old is not sleeping through the night then either they, or you, or both, have a problem. This only perpetuates the myth that if you survive the first year of parenthood your sleep woes will be firmly behind you. Sadly that just isn't the case for most.

If I asked you to guess the average age that most children are able to sleep through the night, what would you say it was?

Six months? Nine maybe? Surely by their first birthday? Research indicates this is not a reality for most children until they reach their second birthday,[1] and in their second year of life 55 per cent are still waking regularly during the night.[2] This information comes as a shock to many of the parents I work with.

Another expectation is that, once children turn one, they should be able to self-soothe themselves to sleep if they do wake at night. Again this is not correct. Research shows that at least 50 per cent of all one-year-olds need parental input in order to help them to settle to sleep.[3] What is perhaps more surprising is that research has shown that, once children reach the age of 18 months, they need more parental help in order to get them to sleep than they did previously.[4] In essence, their sleep *regresses*, yet we expect so much more from them.

So, what is happening during this time frame that causes at least half of all one-year-olds to have such problems sleeping independently? The answer is evident when we consider the daily lives and developments of what I call 'boddlers' (baby-toddlers or new toddlers). A boddler is crossing two worlds. They need us just as much as they did in their first year of life: they are still tiny and relatively helpless and rely on us to fulfil pretty much all of their physical needs – such as hunger, thirst, bathing, changing soiled nappies and dressing appropriately for the temperature. On an emotional level, however, their increasing physical independence – through their new-found abilities to walk, climb and talk – leaves them with a thirst for exploration. I call it the 'me-do-it' phase. It is the job of a boddler to explore the world and learn their own limits. It is our job to keep them safe and provide a secure base for them to return to when the world gets too much. We need to let go just enough: too little or too much can negatively affect their feelings of security. This increasing autonomy is empowering and exciting for boddlers, but it can also be quite terrifying. This is heightened by parents' new expectations for boddlers and utterances such as 'You're a big girl now'. But the fact is they aren't big – far from it, as they constantly battle with conflicting emotions of wanting to be big and wanting to be little. This paradox is a source of great angst for boddlers and their parents, particularly at night-time and at times of separation, such as daytime naps, when our boddler really needs the security of 'being little', through the close proximity of their parents.

The boddlers' new explorations and limit-testing mean that parents inevitably begin to use discipline. Nobody really tends to view a baby as 'naughty', but it is a phrase that is commonly used in reference to a one-year-old, particularly in the latter half of this year. Sadly, a lot of the discipline employed by parents at this time is misguided and involves punishing the child for what is only a natural tendency to explore and have some control over their lives. Traditional discipline techniques, such as time-out and the naughty step, can cause a rift between parent and child that can impact long after the punishment is over, especially if these punishments are conducted in the child's bedroom. One of the keys for easier sleep at this age revolves around what happens during the day. Rather than traditional types of punishment, such as time-out and naughty steps, if we try to respond in a compassionate, empathic way to our children we will preserve our relationship with them and lessen the likelihood of sleep problems as a result. Resetting expectations is vital here: in my previous book *ToddlerCalm* , I discuss what you can realistically expect of a child's behaviour at this age and ways in which to respond that are both fair and firm. You'll find a short summary in the box opposite.

THE COMMON-SENSE WAY OF RESPONDING TO YOUR CHILD'S UNWANTED BEHAVIOUR

Safety: first make sure your child is not in any danger.

Empathy: try to understand the issue from your child's point of view. How are they feeling? How would you like to be treated in a similar scenario? Their brains aren't sophisticated enough at this stage to manipulate.

Naming emotions: helping your child to cope with their big emotions hinges on your child understanding them. A good place to start is by naming the emotion they are feeling: 'I see you are sad that we can't go to the park right now'; 'You are very angry that James wouldn't share his toy with you' and so on.

Support: support your child to cope with the resulting feelings. 'I can see you are very sad. If you like, I'm here for a hug when you need me'; 'Let me know if you would like to go home so you can play with your own toys' and so on.

Exchange: offer your child a safe and acceptable alternative. This shows them that what they are doing is unacceptable, but recognises that they have a need that is unfulfilled: 'I can see you are enjoying making patterns, but it is ruining mummy's lipstick and might stain the wall. Shall we get your paints out instead?'; 'I see you are angry and kicking the cupboard is helping, but that might damage the cupboard, so shall we go into the garden and kick a ball around instead?'

It is important to consider the sheer amount of new physical skills being acquired by the boddler: learning to walk, learning to run, learning to climb, an ever-expanding vocabulary. These new developmental stages are thrilling and exciting for everyone involved, but their acquisition can prove very unsettling for the child. Imagine how much information is passing through their brains at any one point. It must be like attending a week's training that is exhilarating to learn but leaves your head buzzing and feeling like it is going to explode. Understandably, all these new skills can cause boddlers to have unsettled sleep, if only because their brains are constantly buzzing.

SUGGESTED SLEEP ENVIRONMENT FOR A ONE- TO TWO-YEAR-OLD

At this age, creating a good sleeping environment means helping your new toddler to feel comfortable and happy as they take their first steps to independence. Their new-found mobility also means that you need to keep them safe. My suggestions for a good sleep environment at this age are as follows:

- At this age, toddlers may sleep better in their own small bed. This can also help to keep them safe if they have a tendency to climb out of their cot. A special toddler bed can feel cosier to them than a full-size single bed.

- Your toddler is now old enough to have a pillow and duvet, although many still sleep better with a sleeping bag as they have a tendency to kick off their duvet.

- Keep lighting to a minimum at night and the room naturally lit in the daytime.

- Consider using some relaxing alpha music (see page 281) left to play for the duration of the nap time or night.

- Encourage your toddler to sleep with a comforter or favourite cuddly toy, but make sure that you have a spare!

- Ideally your toddler will not have a dummy. If they do, and you are concerned that it is inhibiting their sleep, please see Ellie and Sophia's story on page 189 for ways to wean them off the dummy.

- You can still carry your toddler in a good supportive carrier for nap times if they need to be close to you. Look for a supportive, structured back carrier (for some suggestions see page 280).

What to expect at one to two years

A one-year-old tends to sleep for an average of thirteen hours in any twenty-four-hour period. Around two of these are taken as daytime naps and eleven hours at night. This gives them a split of approximately 85 per cent of their sleep taken at night and now only 15 per cent taken during the day, continuing the trend of moving all of their sleep needs to the night-times. REM sleep drops to around 30 per cent at this age and NREM (quiet) sleep stages are well established. The average sleep cycle lasts around sixty minutes. Over half of all children at this age wake at night and, of those that wake, half will need their parents to go to them to help them settle back to sleep again. They often need parental help with daytime naps too, in order to calm them enough for them to sleep.

At eighteen months it is common for sleep to regress. This does not necessarily mean that the child wakes any more than they did previously; they just need more parental input in order to settle back to sleep, whereas before they may have been more likely to begin a new sleep cycle without alerting their parents that they had woken.

Despite public perception, night feeds remain fairly common, particularly in those children who are still breastfed.

One to two year case study

Sam and Jasmine, twenty-one months

Dear Sarah,

My little girl is twenty-one months and still doesn't sleep through the night. I am exhausted and finding it quite tough. She is still breastfed and wakes several times during the night to feed. She is never awake for long, just feeds and goes straight back to sleep. Whenever we've tried to do anything about it, it has resulted in her waking for longer, being upset, us being even more tired and so we have given up, usually because Jasmine or me has got ill.

Our daily routine goes something like this:

Awake about 7am. My husband is up early for work so this wakes her up most days (at weekends she will sleep until about 8).We have breakfast around 8.30, Jasmine doesn't eat much as she has a big breastfeed when she wakes up so will maybe have a slice of toast. Jasmine has a nap any time from 11.30 that lasts about an hour, longer if she didn't sleep well the night before. Lunch is before or after her nap, or both! Some days she will eat loads, other days barely anything. Yesterday she had two pieces of pasta for example, wouldn't try anything else on her plate even though it was things she normally loves, whereas earlier in the week she had lots of pasta for lunch! Jasmine will normally have an afternoon snack at about 4pm, bread sticks and grapes or a slice of malt loaf for example.

Dinner is normally about 6pm. This is her favourite meal of the day and she will normally eat lots of main course, followed by yoghurt and/or fruit. She breastfeeds on demand during the days I'm with her.

Bedtime routine – bath every couple of days or quiet play after dinner. On the evenings I'm home, I brush Jasmine's teeth, take her upstairs and get her changed into pyjamas. Then I put relaxing music on and breastfeed her to sleep, sat on my bed. Then, when she's asleep, I transfer her to her own bed (she has a mattress on the floor as she hated her cot but moves so much in her sleep she would fall out of a bed). This can take up to an hour.

She then normally sleeps through until about 12–1am when I get into bed with her but will sometimes wake during the evening. During the night, she wakes several times to feed and sometimes won't settle without being permanently attached to my nipple! From 5/6 she is very unsettled and fusses on the boob.

Our daily activities are quite varied:

Monday – swimming in the morning, singing group in afternoon

Tuesday – work alternate weeks, when I work Jasmine goes to my sister who she adores. On these days she doesn't nap as she's too busy having fun with her cousins. My husband collects her, brings her home for dinner and bed

Wednesday – playgroup in morning or quiet time at home, about to start working afternoons

Thursday – take her to my parents in morning then go to work. Parents bring Jas home at some point and have dinner with her and my husband who then puts her to bed

Friday – Jasmine is looked after by my mother-in-law. Husband goes to collect her, they have dinner together and she falls asleep on way home so can be transferred to bed

Saturday – work alternate weeks so if I'm working husband looks after Jasmine or we have a family day. I finish at 5pm so put her to bed.

Sunday – family day

Jasmine used to go to nursery one day a week but was very unhappy there so we stopped. She is now cared for by family, who she loves and she happily waves me off when I leave.

Jasmine's bed is in our bedroom, as we have no alternative until we move house so I think we are all disturbing each other and the three of us are tired! I would describe our relationship as very close, she can be quite clingy and at times will need to be close (attached!) to me. While I absolutely love and adore her, the constantly being needed is draining and sometimes I feel completely 'touched out'.

We have tried taking her to a cranial osteopath for several sessions. This always made her sleep *a lot* more disturbed the first night but there was no noticeable improvement after that. We tried my husband getting her to sleep each night for about a month so it was consistent and she wasn't being fed to sleep but that didn't seem to help.

Jasmine was born ten days late and had meconium in her waters which was making her distressed and her heart rate rise. It was a long labour and the pushing stage was difficult (took about three hours and I had an episiotomy). Fortunately, though, Jasmine has always been healthy so we've had no health worries apart from the normal colds and tummy bugs.

Her sleep has always been very disturbed with lots of waking. It has gradually improved to the point where we are now. I would say she woke hourly when things were really bad. We tried putting her in her cot and leaving her to fall asleep on her own once . . . she screamed and screamed and after twenty minutes I picked her up and promised to never try anything like that again!

We haven't started potty training yet, although she did her first ever wee in the potty yesterday and was very pleased with herself! She has no fears that we know of and doesn't seem bothered when she wakes, sometimes she will just walk over to our bed and wake me up so she doesn't even cry when she wakes up. We have never sent her to her room as a punishment, could never do anything like that to her. She seems to love her bed and has started playing 'going to bed' when we're in the room during the day. We have a lamp on during the evening when she's falling asleep but our room is always quite light thanks to a street light right outside!

My husband has one-to-one time with Jasmine in the mornings while I shower, if she's awake in time! We try and have time when he gets home from work but she finds that transition difficult and often wants to stay with me. Then of course on the days I'm working it's the two of them. They are very close if I'm not around but if I'm there she will always come to me first.

I'm feeling quite stuck with things at the moment, I'm tired but feel too tired to make the effort to change things. Some new gentle ideas and encouragement would be really help-ful. We've had family tell us we need to be more consistent but with the pattern over our week that's not really possible.

Thank you in advance for any advice that you may be able to share with us.
Sam

My BEDTIME solution

The following is a summary of my suggestions to Sam, based on my BEDTIME solution.

Bedsharing/co-sleeping: The current situation with Jasmine sleeping on a mattress on the floor in the parents' bedroom seems like the best one at this time. In the future, Sam may consider trying Jasmine in her own room, though this transition should happen slowly and certainly not when they first move house. Initially, Sam could try sleeping in Jasmine's new room with her for a month or two in order for Jasmine to feel comfortable in her new environment. Sometimes, however, children do sleep better when they have their own sleep space, but obviously Sam will not know what is best for Jasmine until she has the opportunity to try another option.

Expectations: Jasmine's sleeping patterns are very normal and quite common. We know children who breastfeed and bedshare generally wake more at night, which is the case here. It is important to remember, however, that although the number of awakenings is more, often they are easier to handle for both parent and child.

Sam mentions they have tried quite a few things to help Jasmine's sleep, but my concern is their consistency. It is vital that a bedtime routine is adhered to and is identical every night. This is tough when you have been working and are keen for the child to go to sleep. Often parents are inconsistent in their approach, which confuses the child. It's clear that Jasmine's bed-time varies, depending on whether her mother is working or not; for instance, on Friday nights she falls asleep in the car. I suggested to Sam that I felt one of the most important things they should do was carry out an identical bedtime routine every night, no matter who's doing it.

Diet: Jasmine seems to be eating well and I felt it was unlikely her night wakings were related to hunger. Sam works outside of the home a fair amount and perhaps Jasmine's frequent night feeds are related to this. Many children feed at night as a way to reconnect with a mother who has been working in the daytime. This can be a wonderful time for mother and child to feel closer to each other and, if this is the case, then you shouldn't make any changes. Sam refers to being 'touched out', something quite a lot of natural-term, breastfeeding mothers say, and I get the impression that she is ready for their night-time feeding relationship to finish. However, it was important that Sam understood the benefits of this before making her decision.

If Sam wanted to night-wean, I suggested trying to calm Jasmine at night, before offering the breast. If it is obvious that this isn't going to work, which it usually doesn't, then let Jasmine feed, but when she slows and appears to be falling to sleep to take her off the breast. Jasmine is likely to protest, understandably, so I suggested Sam pick a time when life is pretty quiet. I told Sam that if she does decide to try to night-wean then it is really important that Jasmine is not alone; that she should always be with her, offering her comfort. Another option is for Sam to sleep else-where for three or four nights while daddy sleeps with Jasmine and responds at night, which may break the pattern between feeding and returning to sleep. Again, Jasmine probably won't like this, and is likely to cry, so it is important for Sam to remember that Jasmine is never being left alone to cry, and that she will be safe and loved in her daddy's arms. Parent-led night weaning usually doesn't happen without tears. I suggested to Sam that if reading my suggestions was making her uncomfortable then perhaps she wasn't quite ready to night-wean and she may want to revisit it in a few months.

Transitional objects: If Jasmine doesn't have one already, I suggested Sam condition the use of a comforter. Eventually, after at least four to six weeks, Jasmine may associate the comforter with Sam, meaning she'll need her less at night.

IT: Sam doesn't mention if Jasmine watches TV; if she does, I suggested that she has absolutely no TV (or other screen time) for the two hours in the run-up to bedtime, due to its stimulating nature.

Me-time: I always suggest to all parents that they do some serious nurturing work on themselves, even more so if they have a child who wakes regularly at night. Sam is working outside of the house, which means that she does get some valuable head space alone, although it also means that she could be even more tired trying to balance her two lives.

Environment: I suggested to Sam that in the evenings she limit artificial light as much as possible and keep lighting dim. She might also consider using a light in her bedroom that is red-based, or preferably nothing at all. Regarding the street light outside of their bedroom window, I suggested that Sam use a blackout blind, or some blackout window film, to reduce any negative effect it was having on Jasmine.

I also suggested Sam should condition some sound and scent sleep cues, so that Jasmine feels reassured when she wakes after a sleep cycle and can begin a new cycle without Sam's help.

I received the following update from Sam two months after sending her my advice:

Sam's update

Hello Sarah,

Jasmine's sleep is so much better, I feel like a new woman! I decided I wasn't ready to night-wean but decided to stop feeding Jasmine to sleep and this seems to have made a big difference. I feed her downstairs, then she has supper (normally a banana), brushes her teeth and then we go upstairs and I read her stories until she falls asleep. It only took a few nights for her to adjust to this and she now points to my boobs and does her sign for sleeping!

After some trial and error we have settled on an 8pm bedtime which works well for us. We tried the later bedtime that you suggested but it wasn't suitable on the days I work.

Jasmine now normally only wakes about once a night at about 3am, has a quick feed and then kicks me out of her bed! She then sleeps through until the morning. She has even slept through one night, which felt like a miracle! We had a bad spell recently but I think that was due to an outbreak of eczema and she has settled again now the eczema is being treated. I can definitely cope with this for now and may decide to night-wean at a later time but for now it is more than good enough for me.

Thank you for sharing your ideas. There was so much to choose from and some really simple ideas. I took on board your suggestion to cut back on activities and this does seem to have helped. Mostly it was just nice to hear that her sleep was normal and that 'quick fixes' aren't always what they seem.

Many thanks
Sam

Chapter 11

Sleep at two to three years

By the time a child reaches their third year of life the biological differences between their sleep and adult sleep are less noticeable. Children are capable of lasting the night without milk feeds, their circadian rhythms are fairly well established and their levels of REM and NREM sleep are fairly comparable to that of an adult. In theory, this should mean that parents can finally rejoice in a full night's sleep and an easier bedtime. Unfortunately, for many, this is not the case. While, physically, a child is capable of sleep comparable to that of an adult, psychologically, things are very different. From here on in, sleep concerns have a largely emotional cause. And if you have parented a two-year-old you will know quite how emotional they can be!

Many two-year-olds struggle with their autonomy and the insecurities their growing levels of independence and freedom bring. They are definitely caught in the 'wanting to be big and wanting to be little' conundrum on an almost daily basis. Perhaps more pertinent is the constant need for some control over their lives. Most two-year-olds have little or no control over their own lives. Adults decide when toddlers should get up, what they should eat, when they should eat it, where they should go, what they should do (and importantly what they should not do), what they should play with and where and when they should sleep. Toddlers don't like this, understandably. Can you imagine how frustrating it must be to have somebody else controlling every aspect of your life? It's hardly surprising that they rebel against this constant control in the only way that they can – through their behaviour. Refusing to sleep is a great way to try and assert some control. Ultimately, whatever parents do, or don't do, only the toddler can get themselves to sleep. For many toddlers with sleep issues, the underlying problem is not sleep at all, but a toddler desperately crying out for more control over their life.

Toddler control

How can you give a toddler more control? I like to use empathy here: imagine what parts of your life you would be most upset about if somebody else controlled them; for me it would be what I eat and drink and what happened to me on a daily basis. I expect the same would be true for everyone. Perhaps, therefore, your toddler might appreciate you allowing them to have more control over what, how and when they eat. Perhaps they would like more say over their daily routine and where they go, especially if they are tired or under the weather and would rather stay at home. The most important area in which to give your toddler more control, however, is their play. Play is the one part of their lives where toddlers should have full control. They should be allowed to choose what they play with and when they play with it. Too often as parents we direct a child's play: 'Oh darling, you don't want to play with that old thing, play with your new one' or 'Don't be silly, you don't have dinosaurs in a police station, go and get your police figures instead.' We mean well when we do this, seeing it as an educational opportunity, but to a toddler we are encroaching on the one part of their world where they can choose what happens. Allowing our toddlers to have truly toddler-led, free play can have remarkable knock-on effects on all other aspects of their lives, especially sleep. Even better if your toddler invites you to play with them and you allow them to control what you play, too.

Potty training

On a related note, toddlers rarely choose when they get to toilet-train. The decision to begin to ditch nappies is often parent-led, often spurred on by a health professional or by pressure from friends and relatives. If a toddler is not ready to toilet-train there will inevitably be a knock-on effect on their behaviour as they try to assert some of the control that they have lost. Toilet training can be remarkably easy if it is purely toddler-led. When it is parent-led it can prove incredibly stressful, not just for the parent but for the toddler, too. Even daytime toilet training can have a negative impact on sleep, but add night-time toilet training to the mix, with the inevitable bed-wetting that it brings, and things can get tricky. It is perfectly normal for a child to be in nappies at night right up to the age of seven years. Toilet training is always better if it is not rushed and is child-led both day and night.

Arrival of a new sibling

If the power struggles and potty training woes aren't enough, two to three years old is also the most common time for children to have to cope with the arrival of a sibling. Although this can be a wonderful and exciting time for new big brothers and sisters, it can also be incredibly unsettling and can have knock-on effects on every aspect of their behaviour, but particularly sleep.

The unsettling effects of a new baby start early in the pregnancy. If the mother has morning sickness, her behaviour towards her toddler naturally changes as she struggles to cope with the nausea and vomiting and the constant demands of her toddler. As the bump grows and mobility declines, toddlers can be frustrated that they can no longer hug their mother in the same way, and they can be upset and confused when they are told off for climbing over their unborn brother or sister. Moreover, toddlers may be scared of the impact of the new baby, in particular when it comes to their mother's love and attention. Is it any wonder that their sleep can regress at the time when we need ours the most?

The unsettled feelings tend to grow as the birth approaches and toddlers sense the forthcoming change, particularly if we are encouraging them to 'be a big boy' or telling them 'you're a big girl now; there's a new baby coming'. They often don't want to be big, for that means that they are not your baby any more – they are relinquishing that position to a new baby who will get more of your attention and, in your toddler's opinion, your love. They need to be reassured that they are still your baby and reassured that your love for them will not change. Now really is not the time to move to a 'big girl' bed or a 'big boy's' room. These changes should happen very early in the pregnancy or several months after the arrival of the baby, when your toddler feels more confident of their position again.

When the new baby arrives, everything changes and your toddler feels unsure of their place and your affection. They receive far less attention than they did and, when they do receive it, it is often to be told off for waking the baby, touching the baby or accidentally hurting the baby. Some toddlers take this transition in their stride, but for others it can be the most unsettling, scary and upsetting part of their short lives to date. These feelings inevitably lead to sleep problems, particularly at night, when it is dark and scary and your toddler misses your presence. This is heightened if the baby is in your bed or your room and the toddler is alone. For this reason I'm saddened when parenting experts advise parents to shut toddlers in their room, or constantly return them to their room with no eye contact when they wake at night after recently welcoming a new younger sibling. These actions completely ignore the root of the problem and treat the toddler with little respect at a time when they need it most. Empathising with your toddler's feelings and helping them to understand that your love for them has not changed is the key to solving these sleep problems.

There are three points you should always be mindful of in parenting, but these are even more acute when trying to help a toddler to cope with the arrival of a new sibling.

The three Cs

Connection

Most unwanted toddler behaviour, especially sleep related, is due to the toddler feeling disconnected from their parent. If you do one thing regarding your toddler's sleeping and behaviour issues it should be to make sure you work on your connection with them. They need to feel unconditionally loved by you, at all times, but especially when a new sibling has arrived. In my opinion most sleep problems in toddlers, pre-schoolers and older children stem from a connection problem between parent and child. Rebuild that connection and you no longer have a sleep problem. This is why I always recommend parents spend as much one-to-one time with their older child as possible each day, away from the new baby.

Containment

Containment refers to an adult's ability to 'hold' their child's overwhelming emotions. For instance, if the child is scared, the parent is able to help diffuse these fears for the child; if the child is angry, then the parent is calm enough to take these feelings on board from the child and give them back calm feelings in return. If a parent is for some reason unable to take on their child's unwanted emotions, usually because they are too 'full up' themselves, then the child's emotions begin to overrun and erratic, unpleasant behaviour usually follows. The key here is for the parent to nurture themselves enough that they have space to take on their child's feelings. We often get so bogged down in the demands of everyday life – mortgages, bills, work, health concerns, family issues and our own issues and stresses – that we snap at our children because we have no 'space' in our heads for anything else. If our child cannot offload their emotions, they are likely to behave in a negative way, externalising their issues through violent or disruptive behaviour. Sometimes, usually when they are a little older, they can internalise their worries, leading them to become anxious and depressed. Either way, these feelings can lead to huge problems. This is why I continually highlight the importance of adults taking care of their own needs and nurturing themselves, in order that they have space to nurture their children.

Communication

How we communicate with our toddlers is vital. We have to understand that their brains are immature: they don't think like us and they don't behave like us. They are not naughty, they are simply toddlers and we should not punish them for their immature brain development. Instead we need to tailor our communication with them and understand that a lengthy telling-off or explanation of why they must go to sleep are inevitably going to fail. Think about your body language too, and what this is conveying, particularly at night when your toddler is crying for you and you don't look them in the eye or hug them. How do they know that you still love them? Especially when they are waking and crying out for you at night because they don't feel sufficiently connected to you. This is why I always advise parents to respond to their children calmly and lovingly at night, even if it's the last thing you feel like doing. Reconsidering the way you communicate to your toddler, in the daytime and at night, can have a very positive effect on their sleep.

SUGGESTED SLEEP ENVIRONMENT FOR A TWO- TO THREE-YEAR-OLD

At this age concentrate on helping your toddler to feel happy and secure in their sleeping environment. This is particularly important if they have recently become, or are about to be, a big sister or brother.

My suggestions for a good sleep environment at this age are as follows:

- If you haven't yet moved your toddler to a 'big bed' this is the age to do so. If they fall out you could consider using a special bed guard or just putting them on a mattress on the floor.

- If you are going to move your toddler to their own room because of the arrival of a new baby, make sure you do this well in advance of the baby's arrival, or a good few months afterwards, so that they don't feel pushed out by the new arrival.

- Involve your toddler in decorating and choosing items for their room, however much you disagree with their taste. If your toddler loves the items in their room they are more likely to want to spend time in there, however tasteless it may be (in your eyes)!

- At this age, most toddlers can usually cope with a duvet, although you are still likely to find it on the floor in the morning.

- Keep lighting to a minimum at night and the room naturally lit in the daytime.

- Consider using some relaxing alpha music left to play for the duration of the nap time or night.

- Encourage your toddler to sleep with a comforter or favourite cuddly toy, but make sure that you have a spare!

- Consider leaving a beaker of water and a small snack on your toddler's bedside table and leave a few quiet toys out for them to play with when they wake early in the morning. This may buy you an extra few minutes' sleep.

What to expect of your child's sleep at two to three years

At this age, children are sleeping for a total of around twelve hours in any twenty-four-hour period. Eleven hours is taken at night with daytime naps reduced to only one hour in total, which is commonly taken in one block. This means that almost 92 per cent of a toddler's total sleep is taken at night, edging them ever closer to an adult pattern of sleep. Night waking is still common, but toddlers usually settle to sleep fairly quickly after waking.

Two to three year case studies

Lyndsey and Flora, thirty-four months

Dear Sarah,

My daughter Flora (at thirty-four months old) still wakes frequently during the night and it is quite disruptive for the whole family. She has never been what you would call a 'good' sleeper but I'm wondering whether there is anything I can do to help her sleep through the night?

She is a fairly fussy eater, though not abnormally so for her age I don't think. She is obsessed with (cow's) milk and would drink it all day if she could! Otherwise she eats cereal or toast or boiled egg for breakfast, then she'll eat anything from stew and dumplings or spaghetti bolognese to fish fingers and beans or cheese on toast for lunch and supper, with snacks in between (bananas, apples, biscuits, home baking etc.). She will go for days where she just doesn't eat a lot at all, then days where she'll wolf down everything on her plate. When she was tiny I worried that it was food (or lack of it) that was waking her at night, but I now don't believe it has anything to do with her waking.

She has quite serious eczema and has had since she was tiny. I'm sure this was the cause of her waking up a lot during the night between twelve months and twenty-one months (up to three hours awake and itching every night), but funnily enough when her baby sister arrived she started to sleep through, every night, for twelve to thirteen hours! It was amazing, but only lasted two months. I should say we've tried all manner of changes in her diet/clothing/ointments etc. to no avail with the eczema and have settled with a good dermatologist and some steroids for now.

Her birth was fine – great in lots of respects. I was overdue 11 days but went into labour naturally. Labour was long and hard work (approximately twenty hours from start to finish) and I had some diamorphine to get me through it, but nothing else and I delivered vaginally with no complications.

Flora woke frequently from birth as expected, but didn't seem to get any better, apart from the odd six-hour stretch (just teasing me!) she would wake three or four times a night, and by nine months I thought this was 'abnormal' and that she 'should' be sleeping through by now. I was completely exhausted (she was in a cot in her own room). You make all your mistakes with the first-born – I have since done a lot of reading and know a lot better! I had tried leaving her to cry during the daytime from eleven to seventeen weeks. I did this because of family pressure and an understanding, again, that this is what I 'should' do – it was hell, something I regret a great deal, every day. And it didn't work. She was a stubborn little thing (thank goodness) and didn't give in easily – after a while she did get it to a degree, but then we went on holiday and she went right back to square one, so I gave up. I couldn't put either of us through it any more (I never left her at night either – just couldn't bear to). By this time I had stopped feeding her to sleep in the day, so I walked her up and down the road in her buggy to sleep, every sleep, until she was about two! At nine months old I also decided to try and stop feeding her in the night (a friend had done similar). In five nights she was sleeping through, until 5am. She slept like this for three months until her eczema kicked off, at which point she woke up for hours and hours every night (and still got up at 5am!). She would only sleep in her cot, which led to hours and hours of me sitting next to her cot with my arm stretched through the bars, rubbing her back!

She did this pretty much to the day until the arrival of her baby sister aged twenty-one months. Her skin was under control but she was in the habit of needing me a lot. When baby arrived, Daddy tried bedtime and it worked a dream (they let Daddy get away with things they don't with Mummy!). She slept through for a couple of months, 7pm–8am – bliss, and just what I needed with a new baby.

Since then she has regressed to waking up at least once, and often three to four times. I think it started around the same time as she potty trained (though she still wears a nappy at night, she is very aware of her bladder now) and I think she has night terrors?

In terms of our daily routine we are very relaxed. I'm a stay-at-home Mummy, we potter: read books, jump around on the bed, play with toys, paint, go for walks in the woods, jump in muddy puddles. We do the odd singing group at the library and sometimes we go swimming. She also has the occasional day at her granny's house, just down the road, but apart from that she's with me. With her waking at night I try to be as gentle and soothing as possible (hard when her and the baby are screaming in my face and I haven't slept yet!). She still itches a lot so this doesn't help. I hope I have a wonderful relationship with her – she was a clingy baby and toddler for a long time and (apart from the nightmare sleep training) I went with it. She's still fairly attached to me but very independent in certain environments, e.g. Granny's. We are a happy family, we laugh a lot, I would never use her bedroom (or anywhere else) as a place to send her for punishment, though we don't spend a lot of time there.

Daddy now does bedtime routine and he has it down to a fine art – a little TV and cuddle with Daddy on sofa, upstairs for bath, jump around the bedroom (ours), eczema ointment, pyjamas, into her room for stories and milk, kiss goodnight and he leaves her to it. She's brilliant (99 per cent of the time) at going to sleep (though when I do bedtime routine she makes me stay with her, which I don't mind at all). It's dark where we live, so she has a night light.

I love being a stay-at-home Mummy and am very happy with our lives. I am fine emotionally – I've never suffered with PND or anything similar. I have my bad days, I shout when I shouldn't and I am pretty exhausted most of the time! I occasionally have time with the baby and not the toddler, but the only time alone with Flora I have is when the baby is asleep and I try to make as much of this as possible, though sometimes she will also have a little nap on the sofa at the same time. I know it's pretty common for toddlers to wake in the night, but I would love to find a way to help her sleep through the night more often than not. At the moment she wakes at least once a night, every night, often more, at any time – could be 9pm/1am and 3am, or just 1am or 12am and 4am ... she gets out of bed and walks into our room where I co-sleep with the baby (husband usually oblivious in the spare room, though he does try and isn't very patient!). I give her a little milk in her beaker (a 'bad' habit I haven't been brave enough to try and break) and settle her back into bed.

Five minutes and she's normally asleep and we're usually back in bed, except that at least 50 per cent of the time she wakes the baby (a frequent waker and light sleeper). The baby then usually stays awake for an hour or two before going back to sleep, at which point the toddler is often awake again!

It's all a bit of a mess now I see it written down! Part of me just wants to ride it out, in the knowledge that it won't be like this forever, but I would truly love my toddler to be happy enough to sleep all night, but I really don't know what else I can do to gently ease her wakings.

Thanks so much in advance,

Lyndsey

My BEDTIME solution

Here are my suggestions for Lyndsey and Flora, based upon my BEDTIME solution.

Bedsharing/co-sleeping: I suspect Flora wants to come into Lyndsey's room because she knows that the baby is in there too and doesn't want to feel left out. One way of dealing with this is to move her cot into their bedroom as a temporary measure. Or perhaps Daddy could 'room in' with Flora for a while. At least until the baby is in her own room, too.

Expectations: Flora's sleep pattern sounds exhausting, but it is still perfectly normal. A child's sleep doesn't really approach that of an adult's until they are around four years of age, when sleep starts to improve naturally. Children wake regularly throughout the night and some need reassurance to fall back to sleep, and it sounds as if this is part of the issue with Flora.

Lyndsey doesn't mention what time Flora goes to bed, but I wonder if it is too early. We tend to put our toddlers to bed very early in Western society, and if they are not ready to sleep it can often result in more difficult bedtimes. I suggested to Lyndsey that a good natural bedtime would be somewhere around 8 to 9pm.

Lyndsey should stick to a consistent bedtime routine with Flora, as this will have an positive impact on her sleep. It is important that Flora's eczema is kept under control as the discomfort and itching will disrupt her sleep. It is a good idea to incorporate rubbing in Flora's eczema creams into a bedtime massage.

Diet: I asked Lyndsey to consider giving Flora a small supper half an hour to an hour before bedtime, even after her dinner, just in case Flora is waking out of hunger, although I don't think this is the case here. Lyndsey should also be mindful of any additives in Flora's food and could select foods naturally high in tryptophan for Flora's supper (see page 71). I wondered if Flora's cow's milk intake could be related to her eczema and suggested Lyndsey might want to speak to her doctor about this.

Transitional objects: If she doesn't have one already, I suggested Lyndsey condition the use of a comforter for Flora. Lyndsey should cuddle it when she cuddles Flora and involve the comforter in any special time they have together. Lyndsey should also allow Flora to select her own comforter.

IT: I advised Lyndsey that Flora should have absolutely no TV, or other screen time, for the two hours in the run-up to bedtime. Screen time is highly stimulating for children and can inhibit the release of the hormones responsible for sleep, causing disrupted nights. This applies even if the programme is targeted at young children.

Me-time: In order to help Flora still feel connected to Lyndsey I suggested that it would be tremendously helpful for Lyndsey to have 'Mummy and Flora time' every day. This need only be for fifteen minutes, but it does need to be when the baby is not around. I suggested that this might happen when the baby was taking a nap, or perhaps Lyndsey could do this as a priority when Daddy gets in. As much as possible, Lyndsey should let Flora dictate what happens in this time. At weekends, Lyndsey should try to get in an hour's stretch with just her and Flora together for some 'booster time'.

As always, it is vital that Lyndsey nurtures herself too: mothering two small children is hard work!

Environment: I advised Lyndsey that they should spend some time together in the daytime playing in Flora's room. Flora needs to view her room as a lovely, comforting, safe place to be, with good associations. They could play putting her teddies to bed in her cot, read stories, do puzzles and just generally have fun in her room. I suggested that Lyndsey should do this for at least thirty minutes every day.

I advised Lyndsey to swap Flora's night light for a light that is red-based. Light on the white spectrum inhibits the release of sleep hormones, whereas red doesn't. Better still, get rid of the light completely. I also suggested Lyndsey consider using sleep cues, like soft music played constantly. I highlighted the importance of playing the music all night, not just at bedtime. Lastly, Lyndsey might also consider conditioning a relaxing scent such as lavender, in an aromatherapy fan in Flora's bedroom. Again, the scent needs to be present all night.

I received the following update from Lyndsey a few weeks after giving her my tips.

Lyndsey's update

Dear Sarah,

I thought it was about time to give you an update re my toddler's sleeping habits. She has actually gone through a bit of a transformation of late ... I really don't know whether it's your tips or whether she's reached a certain age and is naturally calming down, I suspect a good dose of each.

Anyway, things have been a bit tough as the baby is ever demanding, and Flora's severe eczema has really flared up, so we've been trying all manner of things to sort it out (from oral steroids to getting rid of all detergents in the house!). She's been a very brave girl and somehow her sleep is better, rather than worse.

I changed her night light and added some soft music to her room, which she loves – though I know you said it needed to be on all night, we actually had something in the house which we tried and it certainly hasn't had a bad reaction so we'll keep on with it, though it does switch itself off.

I'm trying very hard to give Flora the attention she needs one-on-one, though it's so hard with a needy, clingy one-year-old who only wants Mummy! When I get the baby to sleep we often spend some time just lying on the sofa and I massage her itchy back or legs – it's lovely and connecting and sometimes she goes to sleep too! If not, we can then play, whatever she wants – painting, baking, reading, whatever, before she helps me with some jobs (she's at the age where this is fun too).

One thing we have done, which I think has made a massive difference, is to spend a good dose of time in her bedroom every day. We really didn't spend a lot of time there before, though I never really thought about it. We go upstairs now at some point every day. I've put her dolls house up there, we get all her upstairs books out and we throw all her teddies on the floor, play, jump on the bed, etc. Now when we go up in the mornings to get dressed after breakfast she often takes herself off into her bedroom to play while I have a shower – it's amazing!

We still have the same bedtime, though (in part due to her eczema) she has a little less TV and longer bath routine. For about two weeks she has regularly been *sleeping through* from 7.15pm until 7.15am *or later*!!!! I can't believe it. It is heaven. She does still wake plenty, and of course we always go to her, but it's not three to five times every single night! She tends to have one or two 'bad' nights a week, where she's up a lot, then one or two nights a week where she's up once, just wants a quick back rub or a quick drink of milk (not been brave enough to swap it for water yet!). But if she is up she tends to catch up the next day (for example, last night she woke about three times before 10pm, husband and I played tag team and I eventually rubbed her back and lay in bed with her), but because she'd had a disrupted evening, she then stayed in bed *the whole night until* 8am!!! On the (fairly regular) nights when she goes through, she has between eleven and twelve hours, and hasn't been up before 6.30am for a while (as I write this I feel the urge to cross all fingers and toes – these things have a habit of coming back to haunt you once you've proclaimed it to the world!). My husband and I have both been downstairs without Flora by about 6.30am to watch the Winter Olympics for half an hour before the day starts (turns out our body clocks are set now!).

I'm so happy and I still can't quite believe how different her sleep is. I really don't mind getting up a bit for her, I'm just so happy she is not consistently waking up every couple of hours – it has really eased things for us all (especially as the baby is still being a bit of a pickle!).

Thank you so much for your advice. It really gave me the chance to think about how we do things and how I can tweak it and it has clearly worked for Flora.

Thanks again, I will be forever grateful.

Lyndsey

Claire and Thomas, two years old

Dear Sarah,

I would very much like your help and advice regarding my two-year-old son's sleep patterns. My partner and I are exhausted after nearly two years of lack of sleep. I honestly cannot remember the last time I had a proper night's rest and this is only getting worse as we now have a thirteen-week-old son who is also nocturnal and seems to survive on very little sleep.

It may be helpful for you to have some background on our situation. Thomas was born at thirty-nine weeks and five days following pre-labour rupture of membranes and subsequent induction of labour. I laboured for several hours and reached maximum infusion rates, which caused hyper-stimulation and a foetal bradycardia resulting in an emergency caesarean section under spinal anaesthetic. Thomas was born in good condition and weighed in at 7lb 2oz.

Everything seemed to be going well and I felt like I was taking motherhood in my stride. Thomas behaved 'normally', feeding regularly doing all the right things and then at around three weeks I felt that he was unwell and following a trip to the GP was told he had a virus. After several subsequent trips to the GP and feeling like I was becoming neurotic (I kept being assured he just had a virus/cold) Thomas had an apnoeic episode and was admitted to the children's hospital and was subsequently diagnosed with Pertussis. He went on to have two further apnoeic episodes. So, for the first six months of his life Thomas spent a lot of time coughing, which was often worse at night-time. I spent a lot of time just watching him sleep and would wake at the slightest movement or lack of movement.

I also have to add that I have never really subscribed to the idea of getting a baby into a 'routine', believing that babies have no concept of routine at such a young age. Also, I didn't want our lives dictated to by a strict bedtime regime. This is something I regret now as my friends' babies all seem to sleep twelve hours whereas Thomas will often be up till 11pm with no sign of sleep in him!

We have tried self-soothing techniques to no avail, we have tried implementing a bedtime routine with little success, I've cut his daytime nap which seemed to worsen the situation, we've bedshared, bed-hopped, moved him back into our room and as a last resort left him to scream, which left me distraught and stressed. The only thing that has worked to a certain extent has been controlled crying. However, it didn't stop the night-time waking and him ultimately ending up in our bed. Thomas talks and often becomes distressed in his sleep. We seem to go a few nights with everything going well and then something will happen, a cold, visitors coming etc. and we are back to square one with him.

An example of a horrendous night was Thomas not settling until 2am. We had put him back to bed numerous times between 8pm and 11pm and in Thomas's eyes this was a game! There was no shouting or anger from us, just gently putting him back to bed each time he got up and stating that it was bedtime. By 2am I was in tears and the baby was waking and restless until 4.30 when he woke for a feed and wouldn't settle after. Thomas was awake at 5.30. I really don't want to shout at Thomas as I don't want to worsen the situation. I myself had horrendous sleep issues until I was ten years old. I stated to my mother '... it's not fair, you and daddy sleep together ...' and I can still see this from a child's perspective. I'm probably being too soft!

Thomas now sleeps in his 'big boys' bed in his own room (initially he was in his cot in his room). The transition from cot to bed doesn't seem to have helped or hindered the situation. We never use his bedroom as 'time out' and have tried to make his bedroom special by decorating it in a pirate theme and involving him in this process. When he does sleep through we praise him endlessly in the hope that this will encourage positive sleep patterns. He did have a plug-in night light which we stopped using as this seemed to make things worse and his twilight turtle only seems to be a source of entertainment rather than an aid to relaxation.

In terms of diet, Thomas has a very sweet tooth, he loves fruit but dislikes vegetables, he also likes dairy and still asks for a bottle of milk. I don't battle with him over food as I know that food is a battle I cannot win, however, I don't allow him to eat only rubbish. Thomas is a very wilful boy and certainly knows his own mind but he is also a very happy boy who charms the birds out of the trees and only has to smile to get his own way! Thomas has been able to work a crowd from a very young age!!! He talks very well and socialises a lot with other children – we rarely have a full day at home and this has been the case from very early on. We attended baby sensory till thirteen months of age, he swims, goes to gym, toddler groups and has play dates with friends as well as walks to parks etc. I absolutely adore Thomas and consider that we have a lovely relationship, with lots of laughs, loves and cuddles and this is only marred by lack of sleep.

I feel constantly emotionally drained and exhausted, I don't feel like I am being a good Mom or partner as I now feel stressed and on the verge of tears most of the time. I also know that this can't be good for Thomas and I can really see a difference in his mood when he has had a good night's sleep.

Sarah, absolutely any help, advice, reassurance that you can offer would be gratefully appreciated.

Claire

My BEDTIME solution

Here are my suggestions for Claire and Thomas, based on my BEDTIME solutions.

Bedsharing/co-sleeping: I suggested that Thomas may be coming into Claire's room as he knows that the baby is in there and he doesn't want to feel left out. One way of dealing with this is to move his bed (or a mattress on the floor) into Claire's room as a temporary measure. Although we may think it is nice for a toddler to have a 'big boy's' room, often their sleep behaviour is really them saying 'I don't want to be a big boy, I'm still your baby'. When Thomas is used to the baby, or the baby moves to his own room, then he can be moved back to his room and is far more likely to stay in there.

Expectations: Thomas's sleep patterns are clearly exhausting, but still normal for a child of his age, especially when a new sibling has joined the family and he is struggling with the feelings that this brings. When we have a new baby we are often guilty of encouraging the older sibling to 'be a big boy', when what they perhaps need the most is our reassurance that they are still our baby, too. Claire mentioned that Thomas has a 'big boy' bed. If the family refer to Thomas's bed as such, this could explain some of his reluctance to sleep in it. Allowing Thomas to 'be a baby' may help him tremendously, and Claire should follow his need and allow him to 'be a big boy' when he wants to be!

On a related point, I suggested that Claire should drop the praise if Thomas sleeps 'well'. Praise is counter-productive for children and, in this instance, I doubt it is helping. If Thomas does sleep 'well', in the morning Claire could say something like 'good morning sleepyhead, you slept a lot last night didn't you? I bet you feel good today', which is much more effective and unconditionally supportive of the child than a comment such as

'Well done for sleeping'. I suspect this unconditional support will really help Thomas, especially since the birth of his brother.

I suggested that Thomas's bedtime may be too early. Some toddlers are naturally night owls and if we try to put them to bed before they are ready, it can often backfire. I suggested Claire try to get Thomas to bed for around 8.30, beginning a good wind-down routine between 7.30 and 8pm.

I was struck by the fact that Claire had tried many things, including a bedtime routine. I find that parents try many things but don't stick to anything for long enough. Gentle sleep techniques require perseverance and consistency, and that means for at least one month, performing the same bedtime routine every night. Often parents give up if, after a week or two, they notice no difference. I suggested that Claire revisit this routine but ensure that it is stuck to rigidly. This is a lot of hard work initially, but consistency for at least a month should result in real change.

Diet: I suggested Claire might consider giving Thomas a small supper of 'slow-burning' carbohydrates, such as toast or porridge, an hour before his bedtime. If she could include foods high in tryptophan (see page 71) in his evening meal this may help too.

Regarding Thomas's sweet tooth, I suggested to Claire that she should be extra mindful of the food that he was eating and the potential impact it might be having on his sleep. Many sweet foods contain artificial colourings, such as tartrazine, which can inhibit sleep, and too much sugar can leave toddlers too stimulated to sleep.

Transitional object: If Thomas doesn't have one already, I suggested Claire should allow him to choose a comfort object, which she should condition him to by always having it around when they are doing something nice together, particularly cuddling.

After a month or so the hope is that Thomas will associate this object with Claire and derive comfort from it when she is not around.

IT: I suggested to Claire that she should limit Thomas's TV and other screen time as much as possible and allow absolutely none in the two-hour run-up to bedtime. Screen time is highly stimulating for children, although it is very easy to rely on the television to entertain an older child when you have younger siblings to attend to. This is counter-productive, however, if it negatively impacts the sleep of the older child.

Me-time: Claire has been through so much with Thomas. I wonder what she is doing for herself and how she feels about her son's birth and early days. I feel that these events may hold some unresolved trauma for Claire and we know that maternal mood has a large impact on child sleep. I asked Claire if she had spoken to anybody in depth about what had happened and suggested that, if she hadn't, it might be a very good idea.

My biggest suggestion for Claire was to really look after herself and try to find some support. Claire sounds like an absolutely wonderful mother, but it's simply not possible for her to look after two small children with such sleep deprivation unless she looks after herself, too. I really did feel that Claire needed some physical and emotional support and suggested she try to form this support network around her as soon as possible.

In addition to some 'me-time', Claire really needs to instigate 'Mummy and Thomas time' each day, for at least fifteen minutes, without Thomas's younger brother around. Initially this may be when the baby is napping during the day. Claire should allow Thomas to control this time together, letting him choose what to do. At the weekend, when Claire's partner is around, ideally this time should increase to around an hour.

Environment: I advised Claire to spend some time with Thomas in the daytime playing in his room. Thomas should form good associations with his room and should view it as a comforting and safe place to be. For this reason it is vital that his room is never used for punishment, such as being sent there if he has done something wrong. Ideally, Claire and Thomas will spend at least half an hour playing in his room every day together. If Claire is short on time she could incorporate this into Thomas's special time with her.

With regards to their days, I suggested Claire should make sure that she gets outside with Thomas for at least fifteen minutes each day around lunchtime. In addition, I suggested that she may try scaling back his activities a little, as their busy days may be over-stimulating for Thomas. I often find if parents have more quiet days at home they have much calmer nights.

In the evenings, once it gets dark, Claire should limit artificial light as much as possible in the home and keep lighting dim. If she has energy-saving light bulbs, she might consider changing them to regular ones in the rooms Thomas spends his evenings in. I also suggested Claire might consider giving Thomas a night light that is red-based, or even better to remove light from his bedroom altogether in the evenings.

Lastly, I suggested Claire might try using sound and scent sleep cues, such as soft music played constantly all night and lavender oil in an aromatherapy fan in Thomas's bedroom. It is important that these sounds and scents are conditioned, for alone they will not work magic. Claire should use the same scent in Thomas's baths and perhaps in a daily massage as part of his bedtime routine. I reminded Claire that she should be consistent, and that it would take at least a month for these cues to be conditioned and produce any noticeable effect.

I received the following letter from Claire a month after giving her my suggestions for Thomas.

Claire's update

Hi Sarah

Thomas's sleep is much better and I think it's for several reasons. Firstly we have relaxed hugely and have accepted that he isn't going to be a twelve-hour-a-night sleeper! He goes to bed around 8–8.30pm which is later than we were trying for before. Bedtime can still be tricky with his delaying tactics but we just go with the flow and that's fine. He gets into bed with us around 4am, which is fine and rather nice as he does fab cuddles, and sleeps till around 7–7.30am.

Illness and visitors always throw a spanner into the works but that's to be expected. I've also realised, as you pointed out, that down-time is good and that the more I do with him the more 'hyper' he can become.

Thank you so much for your help.

Claire

Chapter 12

Sleep at age three to five years

The sleep of pre-schoolers is fairly comparable to that of an adult, especially when considering the percentage of day-time and night-time sleep and REM and NREM phases. By the time a child reaches the age of four, their circadian rhythms are well established and also comparable to those of an adult. Children of this age should not need feeds at night and a grow-ing number have a bladder capacity large enough to see them through the night dry. However, bed-wetting is still very common, affecting around a third of all three- to five-year-olds and many still require nappies at night.

In terms of their physical development and how it affects their sleep, we should be able to expect great things of pre-schoolers. Emotionally, it's a whole other story. This is perhaps one of the most difficult stages for children when it comes to sleeping. Such a lot happens at this age that it is no wonder that a pre-schooler's sleeping patterns can be comparable to that of a young baby. So, what is happening?

Starting pre-school/school

Most children will experience a temporary separation from their parents at this age. This could be starting pre-school at the earlier end of the scale and starting reception at the older end. Many children will take this transition in their stride and positively blossom with their new-found independence, but others may struggle a little.

For those children who struggle with beginning pre-school and infant school, it is understandable that their sleep may suffer as a result and it is often easy for parents to see the link. What is perhaps more difficult to understand is the child who appears to take the transition in their stride and cope well at school, yet still has sleeping problems. Many parents don't see the connection in these cases, although it can definitely exist. Such children may be feeling a disconnect with their parents and need to reconnect with them at night-time after being separated from them all day, or they may have high levels of cortisol during the daytime, due to the stimulating effects of school, and may find it harder to get to sleep at night because of this. Similarly, some children may not cope so well with not being able to take a daytime nap, which leaves them overtired at the end of the day and makes it harder for them to get to sleep.

One of the first things I ask about when I'm contacted by a parent of a three-, four- or five-year-old with sleep problems is how the child is getting on at pre-school or school. Removing as much stress as possible in the daytime can often lead to dramatic improvements in sleep. I sent my first-born son to school part-time (mornings only) until almost the end of his reception year, as he still needed a nap in the afternoon and was too tired to stay at school all day. If he did, he would come home grouchy and overtired and find it very hard to sleep at night. Children do not have to attend full-time schooling until after they are five years old, so if you think it is in your child's best interest to attend part-time then you have a right to request this.

How to stay connected when your child starts school

It is incredibly common for sleep to regress once a child starts school and I often feel this is due to a child needing to feel more connected to their parent. This is often at odds with parents trying to get their children to bed early, desperate that they get enough sleep before another busy day of school, and in an attempt to have an evening to themselves. This can often back-fire and I think one of the best and easiest ways to combat sleep issues with school-aged children is to work on your connection with them and to spend more time together in the evenings. One way to do this is to forget the desire to put them to bed 'nice and early because it's a school night' and push bedtime back a little, in order that the child has more time to connect with you. This may feel like a step backwards, but in almost all cases it will result in the child going to sleep earlier than if you impose a strict early bedtime. For new school starters, I would aim for a bedtime of around 8 to 9pm, beginning the wind-down and bed-time routine no later than 7pm. I have a strict 'no screen time' rule after 7pm and no electrical devices are allowed in bedrooms. I encourage reading and baths after this time.

It is really important to put your child to bed every night, by this I mean going into their bedroom, tucking them in and sitting on the side of their bed for a while. Most children still enjoy a bed-time story, but more important than the story is using this time to really talk with your child. Allowing fifteen minutes every night while your child is in bed and you are sitting or lying next to them is so good for maintaining a connection with them. This is often the time that the child will open up about problems at school or difficulties with friendships and is the best time to discuss these and help them to offload in order to sleep more easily. Making this a part of your family ritual and routine not only at reception age, but in the years that follow, right into the teen years, will help to foster a close connection with your child and help them to feel that you really listen to their worries, fears and anxieties, which, in turn, will make them more likely to talk to you. All of this is also likely to make drifting off to sleep easier for your child.

Nightmares and night terrors

Nightmares and night terrors really come to the fore between the ages of three and five, although some children are affected earlier. Nightmares can be very distressing for both child and parent, since children will often have memories of the nightmare, and for this reason many nightmares can be recurring. I have already suggested some tips that may help nightmares on page 27. Thankfully night terrors are far less common and we can take comfort in the fact that children have no memory of them when they wake. You'll find tips that may help night terrors on page 29.

It is so important to nurture yourself if you have a child suffering from recurrent nightmares and night terrors. In both cases there is not a great deal that can be done to stop the incidences, other than waiting for the child to grow out of them, which they will do. What you can do in the meantime is to look after yourself so that you are less distressed and are more able to look after your child during this difficult period.

Night dryness

Night dryness, or the lack of it, can often be the cause of much conflict between parent and child. It can be incredibly distressing for the child, particularly if they are still wetting the bed with some regularity by the time they start school. I have listed some suggestions to help you to cope with bed-wetting on page 31 and have also listed some support organisations on page 279.

Again, the key to surviving bed-wetting is to take care of your own needs well so that you can be present and, importantly, calm and reassuring, for your child. For so many parents, bed-wetting can descend into a battle with their child, with many taking their child's behaviour personally. This is a time when parent and child need to be as united as possible, not least because bed-wetting can and does have a emotional connection.

The three Cs (and a fourth)

As in the previous chapter, it is really important to foster the 'three Cs' at this age, namely connection, containment and communication. See page 228 for a reminder. I would also add in a fourth C here; one which is important with relation to all child sleep, and parenting in general, but that I feel is extra important in this age range – consistency. It is so important that we are consistent in our approach to our child, being as emotionally available and supportive to them as possible, particularly when five-year-olds go through what I call their 'mini-teenager phase'. It is vital that you stick to whatever BEDTIME plan you implement. Consistency is key and for many parents who have reached this point with ongoing sleep issues with their child, it is often their lack of consistency in approach and actions that has led to their downfall. Stick with a plan and you will eventually notice positive change. You are unlikely to find a magic 'quick fix', and you may have already spent three, four or five years looking for one unsuccessfully, so now may be the time to admit that no such quick fix exists.

What to expect of your child's sleep at three to five years

Total sleep duration in a twenty-four-hour period is now around eleven hours. At the start of this age period, three-year-olds tend to nap for around half an hour per day in the daytime. Almost all five-year-olds have dropped their daytime nap, taking the total percentage of sleep taken at night to almost 100 per cent by the end of this time frame. Night waking is still fairly common, although an increasing percentage are able to get back to sleep without much parental help and the total duration of night waking is now less than five minutes. Sadly, however, almost a third of children in this age range have been on the receiving end of punishment for their sleeping patterns, with over a quarter left to cry themselves to sleep.[1]

Nightmares and night terrors are fairly common for this age bracket, with night terrors affecting around 3 per cent of all three- to five-year-olds and most suffering from nightmares at some point. Bed-wetting is also very common, affecting around 30 per cent of children this age.

SUGGESTED SLEEP ENVIRONMENT FOR A THREE- TO FIVE-YEAR-OLD

At this age, the ideal sleep environment should help your child to feel comfortable, safe, secure and happy. Given that many things change in their life at this stage, perhaps the biggest being starting school, their bedroom should provide them with a safe haven where they can relax.

My suggestions for a good sleep environment at this age are as follows:

- Most children at this age cope just fine in a regular single bed. Don't be tempted to get a cabin or bunk bed yet, as they are still a bit young for these. (I speak from personal experience after my four-year-old fell out of his cabin bed and broke his collar bone.)

- Your child is now old enough to cope well with a duvet, and most children this age will happily sleep with only one pillow, but often they prefer not to use one at all. To an adult this may seem strange and uncomfortable, but it isn't the case for children.

- Keep lighting to a minimum at night, using a red-based night light where possible.

- Keep all technology out of the bedroom. I have a rule that all electronic devices have to stay downstairs between 7pm and 7am. I would never allow my children to have a television in their bedroom as it inhibits sleep too much.

- Consider using some relaxing alpha music or perhaps a special relaxation CD composed specially for young children (see page 281 for recommendations).

- Allow your child to choose the décor and contents of their bedroom, within reason. You may well end up cringing at the super-hero or cartoon-character bedding, but if your child likes it they are far more likely to want to spend time in their bedroom.

> • Don't worry about night dryness. It is very normal for children this age to be in nappies at night. You might consider leaving a potty in their bedroom at night-time for them to use, rather than having to go to the bathroom.

Three to five year case studies

Ally and Ben, age three

Dear Sarah,

Please help! I have a beautiful busy three-year-old boy who I am struggling to get to sleep at night!

It's exhausting me, with having a young baby, and I find myself getting angry, which is not the person I want to be.

I have tried so many different things but would love some ideas on what you may think will work, maybe I just haven't stuck to one thing for long enough?

Ben came into this world a beautiful 8lbs two weeks early. Pregnancy, labour and birth were all great! I was induced two weeks early as I had no amniotic fluid left, I had an epidural which helped a lot and within less than ten hours I had Ben in my arms.

Our first year together was a rocky one – I was a mess! It brings tears to my eyes right now thinking about it. I had severe postnatal depression, although didn't realise until I was recovering from it about seven months after the birth. Not a day went by when I didn't cry. Ben didn't sleep any more than two hours, day and night for the first four and half months. I had lost 27kg and was looking unwell. He had reflux so I slept upright for those four and a half months with him wrapped on me. The next seven months were filled with a lot of rocking, ssshing and some crying it out.

At eight months I returned to work, and since then most weeks are the same. Two or three days at daycare, which he loves, and we go to play group for a morning also. We live in the country so trips in have always taken a wee while. We are kept busy exploring outside, on the farm and at the beach.

Baby number two, who might I add is a breeze, arrived end of July. So since then Ben has had to entertain himself a lot. I feed and cuddle the baby to sleep so that takes up a lot of time. Ben is a good eater, he has his moments but eats a wide variety of veggies, fruit and meat. We bake a lot too, which he loves and he does get some treats. I breastfed until nine months and he only stopped having bottles of milk at two-and-a-half years old.

He toilet-trained himself within a week, two months ago. Awesome stuff! I struggle to deal with his behaviour, although I think he is just a normal energetic toddler and I just need to adapt to that. I struggle with him being so loud and boisterous around our baby, especially during sleep time etc.

There is stress and tension in our house – my partner works huge hours, 5am to 6pm at the moment and I struggle with being a full-time mum sometimes, although I am happy! I look forward to returning to work part time in a couple of months. We have moved house quite a bit which is hard on everyone and are about to again.

So back to the question of can you help me? We have dinner about 5.30 as a family, usually all a little rushed around that time, then the two boys and myself have a bath together and Daddy gets them out and dressed. Then we hang out for a bit, read a couple of books and at 7.15 tell him its nearly bedtime, then at 7.30 we brush our teeth and tuck him into bed, turn on the night light, cuddle him sometimes, read a book or two and from there the fun starts.

He is happy enough in his room but runs in and out of the lounge, turns his room upside down, yells, kicks the walls and is a big excitable mess. We are so exhausted from trying different solutions that we usually end up yelling at him to be quiet and close his eyes followed by threatening to close his door or that he won't get to do something if he doesn't go to sleep. This is terrible I know but we have no idea what to do. Somewhere between 8.45 and 9.30 he will fall asleep. Up until around the time our baby was born we were allowing Ben to jump into our bed when he woke during the night but this got far too hard so we helped him to settle back into his bed, which he seemed happy with.

I hate it and I feel terrible when I go to tuck him in and think to myself how can I get so angry at my little boy? Please help me! Writing this letter to you has broken my heart, how did I turn in to this angry impatient mama and how can I change it? I have completely lost my bond with my little boy since our baby came along and it breaks my heart! I need help to repair this as maybe this is part of the issue? Maybe he doesn't want to sleep as he has no trust in me any more?

Thank you in advance for any further help you can give me.

Ally

My BEDTIME solution

The following sums up the thoughts and suggestions I gave to Ally.

Bedsharing/co-sleeping: Bedsharing with Ben isn't an option for Ally because of the new baby, although 'rooming in' might be. This would involve bringing Ben's bed into their bedroom if there is space or just a mattress on their floor. Alternatively, Ben's dad could sleep in Ben's bedroom for a while to help Ben to still feel connected to his parents at night.

Expectations: Once again, Ben's sleeping sounds exhausting, but normal. Two things strike me here from Ally's letter. Firstly it seems that Ben is naturally ready for sleep at around 8.45. I suggested to Ally that she might consider delaying his bedtime until 8.30pm, a time that seems much more naturally aligned with Ben's body clock. I feel this may be especially important on the days that Ben is in childcare. We know that childcare raises the cortisol levels of children and they need some time in their own home environment with their parents in order for these levels to drop enough for them to sleep, and the same may also be true for Ben when he is at pre-school.

Second, it's great that Ally has an evening routine, but it seems to last for two hours, which is too long, and may be quite disjointed. I suggested that they may spend some time as a family, playing, after dinner and begin Ben's bedtime routine with his bath, around an hour before they want him in bed, moving straight onto tooth brushing, cuddles and story time. I felt this would give Ben much stronger expectations of bedtime.

It's really important that Ally keeps to the same routine at weekends; she shouldn't be tempted to try for an earlier or later night, or skipping part of the bedtime routine, as this will throw Ben's body clock and expectations out of sync.

Lastly, I suggested that when Ben does wake at night, Ally should always be there for him and reassuring, never threatening to shut his door or take away special treats. If Ben struggles to get back to sleep, or indeed fall asleep in the first place, Ally could encourage him to lie next to her, but tell him she is tired so is going back to sleep, and she should then lie with her eyes closed. She can encourage Ben to do the same as her and indicate that if he is not ready to sleep that that's OK, he can just lie and relax next to her. This shows Ben that his parents are still there for him, but models good sleeping behaviour to him.

Diet: I wondered if Ally had ever considered that Ben may have any food allergies, such as cow's milk protein. This could be impacting on his sleep and may well be the cause of his earlier reflux, too. I also suggested that Ally might consider giving Ben a small supper half an hour before his bedtime, just in case he is waking due to hunger.

Transitional object: If Ben doesn't have one already, I suggested Ally might arrange a special trip to buy one and then spend some time conditioning it in order that Ben may take comfort from the object and link it with Ally.

IT: Ally doesn't mention that TV forms part of her evening routine, but just in case I highlighted that Ben should have absolutely no screen time in the two hours leading up to bedtime.

Me-time: I suggested that there were two things Ally might like to work upon. The first is taking care of herself, considering that she spends twelve hours per day, five days a week caring for two small children completely on her own. The second issue I think she would really benefit from working on is her relationship with Ben. I feel that if she builds on the connection with him that his behaviour, including his sleep, will dramatically improve. Add to this Ally will be able to heal the bond between her and her son, which will help her emotional well-being and may in turn have an even more positive knock-on effect on Ben's behaviour, both in the day and at night.

I suggested that Ally should arrange a special 'Mummy and Ben time', which she can do either while the baby sleeps or immediately Ben's dad gets home from work at night. This should be for at least fifteen minutes, but really as long as Ally can spare. She should spend this time really working on her bond with Ben, playing games led by him and reassuring him how much she loves him. It would be amazing if she could spare a whole Saturday or Sunday every now and again to spend a day with Ben somewhere away from the baby, to really 'fill him up' with her love. This wouldn't just benefit Ben, but Ally too.

Environment: I advised Ally to spend at least half an hour every day playing in Ben's bedroom. Ben should view his bedroom as a safe and comforting sanctuary with many good memories. He should never be shut in his room, or threatened with this, as this associates his bedroom with punishment and fear, which naturally will result in him not wanting to be in there.

I also suggested that Ally should ensure Ben gets at least fifteen minutes outside every day around lunchtime. When night falls, Ally should limit artificial light as much as possible in the home and keep lighting dim. If she has energy-saving light bulbs she might consider changing them to regular ones in the rooms they spend the hours between 5 and 7pm in. I also suggested Ally should either remove all light from Ben's room or switch any light that is in there to a red-based one.

Lastly, I suggested Ally use multi-sensory sleep cues, like relaxing music, or perhaps even a special relaxation CD composed for children, and a relaxing scent, such as lavender, as part of Ben's bedtime routine. The CD and smell should be present all night, or at least Ben should have easy access to the CD player and fan in order to turn them on himself when he wakes at night and needs familiar comforters to return to sleep.

Sarah and James, age four

Dear Sarah,

My little boy is four and for the last ten months or so has been suffering from what I think are 'night terrors'. We now have a newborn and are finding it difficult to comfort our boy while meeting the baby's needs. We also have an eight-year-old girl.

These night terrors happen up to three times per week, once or twice a month. So it is not every night but they do tend to happen in clusters. It is usually around midnight but on occasion has been up to 2am. They can last on average twenty minutes but have been up to 45 minutes and have, at times, reoccurred ten minutes later.

During this time James will wake up shouting 'no no no, agh', then sometimes he will call for one of us but not always. We go to him straight away. He can be very angry towards me if I go and not so much to his dad. We try to reassure him saying 'Shush honey, Daddy's here, Mummy's here, you're safe, there's nothing nasty.' We use his name and speak softly, repeating ourselves. He doesn't say words, it's mainly shouting noises like a rage, a temper. It's really loud. He will say no and kick his duvet off. He thrashes on the bed, throwing himself to the bottom of the bed and sometimes clearing out all his teddies and sippy cup of water.

I'll kneel on the floor offering my lap, my arms saying 'hush do you want a cuddle? Mummy's here.' Eventually he will calm and almost collapse into me. He will go back to bed and I stroke his head to reassure him as he calms.

I find these episodes upsetting emotionally for me but also to see him so distressed. What causes this? How can I help him and help it go away? Towards the end of my pregnancy my husband would go more than me as he could stay calmer and James's kicks would be quite forceful.

This started last year around February and was particularly bad in March when his dad was away for two weeks. It continued all year, and in October/November he had a few which his dad handled as I was feeding baby. It has improved this last month. He goes to bed around 7 to 8pm and is asleep by half past. I check him around 9. If he wakes it is around 11, but has been 2am. He wakes for the day at 7am very happy and full of energy.

Up until a week ago he slept in a junior bed that was his cot bed. We have just bought him a single bed mid-sleeper. He has been waking at 3 to 4am but wide awake and asking for the toilet. In November my husband gave him a pillow and this seems to have helped and I read somewhere to put socks on! He has been in his own room since eight to nine months old.

On Monday and Tuesday he goes to my aunt's nursery, which is only small with no more than six children under four. She does have some before- and after-school children. My mum is her assistant, and his cousins also go.

He has always been with me on Wednesday and is at my mum's on Thursday and with his Nana on Friday. Since September he has started a local pre-school Wednesday and Thursday mornings only, with children he will go to primary school with, and since September I have been at home on maternity leave. Weekends we are all at home together.

My relationship with James is very close and fun. We have a strong bond. He is also close to his dad and his big sister. We tried gently persuading James out of nappies from about two-and-a-half. It wasn't until a week after the baby was born that he took control, asked to use the toilet and was dry (in the past when we tried it he was very wet and unaware). At three-and-a-half he will have accidents if engrossed in playing but is getting more independent, even getting clean clothes. This last week when we have calmed him from crying out at night he has asked to go to the toilet each time and his pull-up has been almost dry.

He has no obvious fears. He likes super hero and baddie play, dragons, dinosaurs, Star Wars, pirates, Power Rangers. He plays out dressing up and small world play with Lego and figures. He has been fearful of 'noise' machines such as hand dryers in public toilets, hair dryers, Hoovers and food processors. As he gets older he is using his language to be rational about these noises and what makes them.

James always has a story before sleep that he chooses and he has favourites, he likes to choose a song with the light off and then hugs and kisses, he chooses how many. We tell him he is safe and where we will be and that we love him and are looking after him. You then hear him talking to teddies and he falls asleep. He likes bedtime.

Emotionally I have been concerned that I have done something wrong. Has the day been too busy or not busy enough? Is it because he didn't handle a situation during the day? Is he stressed or unhappy about something and couldn't express himself? Despite having extremely well developed language he can struggle to get his words out when in a temper. I get upset when he cries and rages at night. I carry it on my shoulders. My husband stays incredibly calm for him. He will swear when he gets back into bed though, after it's all calm!

Look forward to hearing from you.

Sarah

My BEDTIME solution

The following is a summary of my suggestions for Sarah and her family.

Bedsharing/co-sleeping: I didn't think this was relevant in this case. James seems settled where he is.

Expectations: I suggested to Sarah that in my opinion this did sound very much like night terrors. I reassured her that these were not a result of anything she had or hadn't done and certainly nothing to blame herself for. I highlighted that night terrors are fairly common for children of James's age and confirmed that in most cases there are no obvious causes. Although some link night terrors to periods of stress and upheaval and being overtired, I reassured Sarah that I didn't think any of these applied in her son's case. I told Sarah that in many cases night terrors are just strange blips in a sleep cycle that affect boys more than girls and that children usually grow out of them by around five years of age.

I reassured Sarah that although night terrors occur in a stage of sleep where it may seem as if James is awake, he isn't; he's very much asleep, even though sometimes children with night terrors can appear quite lucid. This is good news for James, as he will have no recollection of the events or suffer any trauma from them.

Lastly, I reassured Sarah that she was doing the right things when James has a night terror. The key is about keeping him as safe as possible until it subsides and he naturally grows out of them.

I mentioned the Lask protocol of dealing with night terrors (see page 29). Sarah mentions that the events occur commonly at midnight. If she can spot a pattern she should wake James fully fifteen minutes before the usual time the terrors happen and keep him awake for ten minutes. This interrupts the sleep cycle and in most cases prevents it from happening.

Diet: I suggested Sarah may want to look at James's diet for any potential triggers, just in case she can spot a link between any specific food intake and his night terrors.

Transitional object: I didn't think this was particularly relevant here.

IT: I suggested that Sarah limit James's screen time as much as possible, particularly in the evenings in case this was having an effect on his sleep cycles.

Me-time: I suggested Sarah could try to make sure she has special 'one-to-one' time with James for fifteen minutes every day, which benefits every child, particularly those with siblings. I did mention, however, that I didn't think James's night terrors were related to anything she is or isn't doing.

Sarah already encourages James to talk about any fears and concerns, which is great. Another option could be to introduce books into James's story time that deal with any worries he might have. I feel that the most important point in this case is that Sarah looks after herself. Night terrors are incredibly traumatising for a parent to watch, feeling helpless. Sarah needs to keep reminding herself of what a great mother she is and take plenty of time to relax and care for her own well-being, as well as that of her children.

Environment: I suggested that Sarah keep James's room dimly lit, with a red night light to reassure him when he wakes, if he would like one. I also suggested that she may want to try a relaxation CD with him, to listen to in the run-up to bedtime, to ensure he goes to sleep as calmly as possible.

After sending Sarah my suggestions for helping James's night terrors, I received the following response from her.

Sarah's update

Hi Sarah,

As I read your reply James had a huge night terror. Shouted at me saying 'Mummy you do things wrong' and he picked up toys and launched them across the room. He was the angriest I have ever seen him. He screamed he needed a wee so I took him to the toilet, then he went back to bed and was fast asleep. Wow! My back is killing me and I feel exhausted. I can't believe he can be so irrational and emotional and asleep. I will start a diary of this just to see.

Cheers Sarah

I replied, reassuring Sarah that she was doing the right things and telling her not to take James's behaviour personally. I suggested that James's night terrors would not last for long and the important thing was for Sarah to be kind to herself during this time. She replied a week later with the following:

I just wanted to say thank you for replying to my email last week, for listening and understanding. It was a particularly hard week last week. Juggling three little ones is not for the faint hearted (eight-year-old girls have many emotions).

James has slept really well the past four nights. Acceptance of no consistency for sleep is the way to stay calm. Thank you again, it meant a lot to me during a down period of time.

Kind regards
Sarah

Chapter 13

Summary and sleep action plan

In this final section of the book, I summarise all the points I have covered in previous chapters, to enable you to formulate your own plan of action for your family, based on my BEDTIME solution. I have come to realise over the years that many parents would very much like me to tell them exactly what to do to solve their child's sleep problems. However, I have issues with this on many levels. First, if I told you exactly what to do this would be disempowering for you, and my aim with all my work is to empower parents to understand their children and to be able to formulate their own solutions by being their own best experts. Second, I am at a significant disadvantage to you, having never met your child or had insight into your family dynamics, so if I gave you a rigid step-by-step sleep plan for your child it would be naïve at best and useless, if not damaging, at worst. Lastly, children change quickly and parents need to adapt their approaches, therefore by empowering you to formulate your own plan of action you will easily be able to do this a few months down the line, or even in a couple of years with a different child.

If you turn to pages 275–78 of this book, you will find some blank pages featuring the headings from my BEDTIME points. The purpose of these pages is for you to work through your unique scenario, and write down your own seven-point action plan, by carefully considering each BEDTIME point in turn. This will give you a comprehensive sleep plan that is unique to your family.

The last point I would like to emphasise here is the issue of consistency and patience. I know how tempting the idea of a 'quick fix' is when you are desperate for sleep. Quick fixes rarely work in the long term though, or at least not without a significant price. As the saying goes, 'there are no short cuts to any place worth going'. Many of my suggestions involve conditioning sleep cues and it takes time to build up the associations. In all cases, I advise giving your plan a minimum of six weeks of consistent, daily action before assessing results. I cannot emphasise enough how important this point is.

While it may seem daunting to spend the next six weeks dramatically reassessing your daily life and home environment, it will bring untold benefits to your child and to you – some of which may never have occurred to you when you sought out a gentle sleep solution. I hope you will be pleasantly surprised at all of the positive side effects.

Here is a brief summary of the points to consider.

Bedsharing/co-sleeping

- How do you feel about sharing a bed with your child if it is safe for your situation?

- If you are considering bedsharing now, make sure you are aware of all of the safety guidelines. See page 97.

- How do you feel about co-sleeping or 'rooming in'? Is this possible? How might you make this work in your room?

- Can your partner 'room in' with your child in their room for a while?

- If you are hoping to move your child out of your bed or your room see pages 99–101.

Expectations

- Are your expectations of your child's sleep realistic? How do they compare with the norms of sleep of a child the same age?

- Is your child's bedtime appropriate for their age? Is it possible you may need to delay it?

- Are you giving your child at least two hours at home after daycare before beginning the bedtime routine, to allow time for their cortisol levels to fall sufficiently?

- Have you considered the impact of your child's daily activities on their sleep?

- Does your child have a wind-down and bedtime routine (lasting a minimum of half an hour) that is followed consistently each and every day?

- How can you add to your child's wind-down and bedtime routine to help them form appropriate expectations?

- Does your child have a nap-time routine? Is this followed consistently every day and by everybody who cares for your child?

Diet

- If you are breastfeeding your baby, have you visited a lactation consultant or breastfeeding counsellor to check their latch and for tongue/lip tie?

- If your baby is formula-fed, have they been checked for tongue/lip tie?

- Is it possible that your child may have an allergy or intolerance that is affecting their sleep?

- Does your child eat too much sugar or too many food colourings and additives?

- Can you give your child more food that is high in tryptophan (see page 71)?

- Have you tried giving your child a small supper half an hour to an hour before bedtime?

- Consider giving your child an omega-3 supplement every day.

Transitional objects

- Does your child have a comfort object already? If not, can you let them choose one (or select one for them if they are too young) and begin to condition a link with you, in order that in time they associate the object with you and take comfort from it?

- If your child has a particularly loved comforter, try to get hold of a second identical one in case the original is lost.

- Ensure that your child can easily access the comforter, particularly at night-time.

IT

- Does your child spend too much time in front of a screen? Turn off the television two hours before you want your child to go to sleep and limit daytime screen exposure as much as possible.

- Make sure that there is nothing on television that is causing fear for your child.

- Never have a television in your child's bedroom and consider banning other screens too.

Me-time

- What do you do to look after yourself? How can you nurture yourself more?

- How do you feel about your child's birth? Do you have unresolved feelings and could you benefit from speaking to somebody about them?

- How much support do you have? How can you get more?

- How much one-to-one time do you have with your child? Ensure that you have around half an hour of 'special time' per child per day, more at weekends if possible.

- Consider a special 'booster' session of 'special time' for older children, all day Saturday or Sunday, particularly if you feel that your connection with them is not as strong as it could be.

- Do you spend fifteen minutes chatting with your older child after you have put them to bed?

Environment

- Do you get outside with your child every single day around lunchtime or the early afternoon to expose them to natural light?

- Do you keep lighting dim in the evening when night falls?

- Do you have energy-saving light bulbs that could be replaced with red light bulbs in rooms where your child spends the most time in the evening?

- Can you remove the light from your child's bedroom at night-time completely? If not, consider changing the light source to a red bulb.

- Do you spend time together playing in your child's room in the daytime, helping them to view it as a happy place? (Remember, never send your child to their room or shut them in in an attempt to discipline them.)

- Can you incorporate a scent cue, such as lavender oil in a battery operated fan? Remember this should be conditioned first (see page 112).

- Can you incorporate a sound cue, such as relaxing music or white noise? Remember this should be conditioned first and should be present all night.

- Can your older child wind down with a relaxation CD?

- Do you have story time every night? Can you select books related to your child's concerns to help them to cope better?

- For older children, have you let them have some control over what is in their bedroom?

- If your child is experiencing nightmares have you considered making some 'monster spray' (see page 28), using a dream catcher or giving them a toy to take care of at night?

Parental sleep plan: BEDTIME

Bedsharing/co-sleeping

Expectations

Diet

Transitional objects

IT

Me-time

Environment

Resources

Gentle Sleep Book website www.gentlesleepbook.com

Gentle Parenting Website www.gentleparenting.co.uk

Doula UK Postnatal Doulas www.doula.org.uk

Homestart Family Support www.home-start.org.uk

Lactation Consultants of Great Britain www.lcgb.org

General Osteopathic Council www.osteopathy.org.uk

British Chiropractic Association www.chiropractic-uk.co.uk

Infant Sleep Information Source www.isisonline.org.uk

Evolutionary Parenting www.evolutionaryparenting.com

Mother–Baby Behavioural Sleep Laboratory
www.cosleeping.nd.edu

Lullaby Trust www.lullabytrust.org.uk

Babywearing UK www.babywearing.co.uk

Recommended products

Slings for younger babies

Boba www.boba.com

ByKay www.bykay.com

Close Baby Carrier www.closefamily.com

Je Porte Mon Bebe www.jeportemonbebe.com

KariMe www.kari-me.com

Moby Wrap www.mobywrap.com

Carriers for older babies and toddlers

Beco www.becobabycarrier.com

Boba www.boba.com

ByKay www.bykay.com

Connecta www.connectababycarrier.com

Manduca www.manduca-baby-carrier.eu

Tula www.babytula.com

Co-sleeper cribs

Arm's Reach www.armsreach.com

Bednest www.bednest.com

Snuzpod www.thelittlegreensheep.co.uk

Sleep cues

Gentle Sleep Music for Babies and Gentle Sleep Music for Toddlers from www.itunes.com and www.amazon.co.uk

Battery operated aromatherapy fan from www.bodi-tek.co.uk

John Levine's Alpha Music www.silenceofmusic.com

Relax Kids Relaxation CDs from www.relaxkids.com

Steven Halpern's Alpha Music www.innerpeacemusic.com

Toiletries for bedtime routines

Night Night Balm www.badgerbalm.com

Weleda Relaxing Lavender Bath Milk www.weleda.co.uk

Weleda Lavender Relaxing Body Oil www.weleda.co.uk

Transitional objects

Cuski Baby Comforter www.cuski.com

Swaddling

Cuski Bamboo Swandoodle www.cuski.com

Love to Dream, Love to Swaddle Up www.cheekyrascals.co.uk

Bedtime books to share with your child

Paul Czajak, *Monster Needs his Sleep*, Scarletta Press (2014)

Ed Emberley, *Go Away Big Green Monster*, Little, Brown (1993)

Jen Green, *I'm Important Too*, Wayland (2007)

Katherine Havener, *Nursies When the Sun Shines*, Elea Press (2013)

Virginia Ironside and Frank Rodgers, *The Huge Bag of Worries*, Hodder (2004)

Jenni Overend, *Hello Baby*, Frances Lincoln (2009)

Margot Sunderland and Nicky Armstrong, *Teenie Weenie in a Too Big World*, Speechmark Publishing (2003)

Jill Tomlinson, *The Owl who was Afraid of the Dark*, Egmont (2014)

Martin Waddell and Barbara Firth, *Can't you Sleep Little Bear?*, Walker (2013)

Bibliography

Australian Association of Infant Mental Health. Position Paper
1: Controlled Crying. Issued November 2002; revised March
2004. www.aaimhi.org/inewsfiles/controlled_crying.pdf

John Bowlby, *A Secure Base*, Routledge (2005)

Dana Breen, *Talking with Mothers*, Free Association Books
(1989)

Judy S. DeLoache and Alma Gottlieb, *A World of Babies:
Imagined Childcare Guides for Seven Societies*, Cambridge
University Press (2000)

Roger Ekirch, *At Day's Close: Night in Times Past,* Pheonix (2005)

Carol Garhart Mooney, *Theories of Attachment: An Introduction
to Bowlby, Ainsworth, Gerber, Brazelton, Kennell, and Klause*,
Redleaf Press (2009)

Jerry Holmes, *John Bowlby and Attachment Theory*, Routledge
(1993)

Deborah Jackson, *Mother and Child: The Secret Wisdom of
Pregnancy, Birth and Motherhood*, Duncan Baird Publishers
(2001)

Deborah Jackson, *Three in a Bed: The Benefits of Sleeping with
your Baby*, Bloomsbury Publishing (2003)

K. Kendall-Tackett and W. Middlemiss, *The Science of Mother Infant Sleep*, Praclarus Press (2013)

Melvin Konner, *Childhood: A Multicultural View*, Little, Brown (1992)

J. McKenna, *Sleeping with your Baby: A Parent's Guide to Cosleeping*, Platypus Media (2007)

Dr John Maltby, *Personality, Individual Differences and Intelligence*, Pearson (2013)

Alan Slater and Gavin Bremner, *An Introduction to Developmental Psychology*, John Wiley and Sons (2011)

Naomi Stadlen, *What Mothers Do: Especially When it Looks Like Nothing*, Piatkus (2005)

Melanie Waxman, *Bless the Baby: A Wise Mother's Book of Protective Prayers, Rituals, Devices and Worldly Wisdom*, Carroll and Brown (2001)

On the web

Colour wavelengths and melatonin, Debra Skene, University of Surrey:
http://www.nature.com/nature/journal/v497/n7450_upp/full/497S10a.html?WT.ec_id=NATURE-20130523

Eight-hour sleep, Gregg Jacobs:
http://www.bbc.co.uk/news/magazine 'The myth of the eight-hour sleep', 22 February 2012

Energy-saving light bulb:
http://en.wikipedia.org/wiki/Energy_saving_lightbulb Accessed 14/02/2014

Government statistics on childcare and early years education: http://www.statistics.gov.uk/hub/children-education-skills/children-and-early-years-education/children-at-childcare Accessed 14/02/2014

'In arms parenting: a history and cultural education', Barbara Wishingrad: http://nurturingacrosscultures.org/us/articles/87-in-arms-parenting-a-history-and-cultural-education.html Accessed 18/02/14

Infant Sleep Information Source, University of Durham: http://www.dur.ac.uk/resources/isis.online/pdfs/ISISPDFSlings July2013.pdf
Accessed 18/2/14

Sleep apnoea: http://www.gosh.nhs.uk/medical-conditions/search-for-medical-conditions/sleep-apnoea/ Accessed 14/02/2014

References

Introduction

1   Armstrong, K. L., Quinn, R. A., Dadds, M. R., 'The sleep patterns of normal children', *Med J Aust.*, 161(3) (1994), pp. 202–6.

2   Chung, M., Oden, R. P., Joyner, B. L., Sims, A., Moon, R. Y., 'Safe infant sleep recommendations on the Internet: let's Google it', *J Pediatr.*, 161(6) (2012), pp. 1080–4.

Chapter 1

1   Mirmiran, M., Maas, Y. G., Ariagno, R. L., 'Development of fetal and neonatal sleep and circadian rhythms', *Sleep Med Rev.*, 7(4) (2003), pp. 321–34.

2   Antonini, S. R., Jorge, S. M., Moreira, A. C., 'The emergence of salivary cortisol circadian rhythm and its relationship to sleep activity in preterm infants', *Clin Endocrinol.*, 52(4) (2000), pp. 423–6; McGraw, K., Hoffmann, R., Harker, C., Herman, J. H., 'The development of circadian rhythms in a human infant', *Sleep*, 22(3) (1999), pp. 303–10.

3   Mirmiran, M., Maas, Y. G., Ariagno, R. L., 'Development of fetal and neonatal sleep and circadian rhythms', *Sleep Med Rev.*, 7(4) (2003), pp. 321–34.

4   Marks, G. A., Shaffery, J. P., Oksenberg, A., Speciale, S. G., Roffwarg, H. P., 'A functional role for REM sleep in brain maturation', *Behav Brain Res.*, 69(1–2) (1995), pp. 1–11.

5 Blair, P. S., Humphreys, J. S., Gringras, P., Taheri, S., Scott, N., Emond, A., Henderson, J., Fleming, P. J., 'Childhood sleep duration and associated demographic characteristics in an English cohort', *Sleep*, 35(3) (2012), pp. 353–60.

6 Touchette, E., Dionne, G., Forget-Dubois, N., Petit, D. et al, 'Genetic and environmental influences on daytime and nighttime sleep duration in early childhood', *Pediatrics*, 131(6) (2013), pp. 1874–80.

7 Matricciani, L. A., Olds, T. S., Blunden, S., Rigney, G., Williams, M. T., 'Never enough sleep: a brief history of sleep recommendations for children', *Pediatrics*, 129(3) (2012), pp. 548–56.

8 Blair, P. S., Humphreys, J. S., Gringras, P., Taheri, S., Scott, N., Emond, A., Henderson, J., Fleming, P. J., 'Childhood sleep duration and associated demographic characteristics in an English cohort', *Sleep*, 35(3) (2012), pp. 353–60.

9 Price, A. M., Brown, J. E., Bittman, M., Wake, M., Quach, J., Hiscock, H., 'Children's sleep patterns from 0 to 9 years: Australian population longitudinal study', *Arch Dis Child*, 99(2) (2014), pp. 119–25.

10 Powell, S., Kubba, H., O'Brien, C., Tremlett, M., 'Paediatric obstructive sleep apnoea', *BMJ*, 340 (2010).

11 Zisenwine, T., Kaplan, M., Kushnir, J., Sadeh, A., 'Nighttime fears and fantasy–reality differentiation in preschool children', *Child Psychiatry & Human Development*, 44(1) (2012), pp. 186–99.

12 Lask, B., 'Novel and non-toxic treatment for night terrors', *BMJ*, 297(6648) (1988).

13 Ibid.

14 Fergusson, D. M., Horwood, L. J., Shannon, F. T., 'Factors related to the age of attainment of nocturnal bladder control: an 8-year longitudinal study', *Pediatrics*, 78(5) (1986), pp. 884–90.

Chapter 2

1 Czeisler, C. A. 'Perspective: casting light on sleep deficiency', *Nature*, 497(7450) (2013).

2 Wright, K. P. Jr, McHill, A. W., Birks, B. R., Griffin, B. R., Rusterholz, T., Chinoy, E. D., 'Entrainment of the human circadian clock to the natural light–dark cycle', *Current Biology*, 23(16) (2013), pp. 1554–8.

3 Holzman, D. C., 'What's in a color? The unique human health effects of blue light', *Environ Health Perspect.*, 118(1) (2010), pp. 22–7.

4 Warman, V. L., Dijk, D. J., Warman, G. R., Arendt, J., Skene, D. J., 'Phase advancing human circadian rhythms with short wavelength light', *Neurosci Lett.*, 342 (2003), pp. 37–40.

5 Foley, L. S., Maddison, R., Jiang, Y., Marsh, S., Olds, T., Ridley, K., 'Presleep activities and time of sleep onset in children', *Pediatr.*, 131(2) (2013), pp. 276–82.

6 Nuutinen, T., Ray, C., Roos, E., 'Do computer use, TV viewing, and the presence of the media in the bedroom predict school-aged children's sleep habits in a longitudinal study', *BMC Public Health*, 13(1) (2013), p. 684.

7 Kurdziel, L., Duclos, K., Spencer, R., 'Sleep spindles in midday naps enhance learning in preschool children', *Proc Natl Acad Sci USA*, 110(43) (2013), pp. 17267–72.

8 Vermeer, H. J., Ijzendoorn, V., Marinus, H., 'Children's elevated cortisol levels at daycare: a review and meta-analysis', *Early Childhood Research Quarterly*, 21(3) (2006), pp. 390–401.

9 Lahti, T. A., Leppämäki, S., Lönnqvist, J., Partonen, T., 'Transitions into and out of daylight saving time compromise sleep and the rest–activity cycles', *BMC Physiology*, 8(3) (2008).

Chapter 3

1 Burdakov, D., Jensen, L. T., Alexopoulos, H., Williams, R. H., Fearon, I. M., O'Kelly, I., Gerasimenko, O., Fugger, L., Verkhratsky, A., 'Tandem-pore K+ channels mediate inhibition of orexin neurons by glucose', *Neuron.*, 50(5) (2006), pp. 711–22.

2 Naska, A., Oikonomou, E., Trichopoulou, A., Psaltopoulou, T., Trichopoulos, D., 'Siesta in healthy adults and coronary mortality in the general population', *Arch Intern Med.*, 167(3) (2007), pp. 296–301.

3 Mindell, J. A., Sadeh, A., Kwon, R., Goh, D. Y., 'Cross-cultural differences in the sleep of preschool children', *Sleep Med.*, 14(12) (2013), pp. 1283–9.

4 Worthman, C. M., Melby, M. K., 'Toward a comparative developmental ecology of human sleep', *Adolescent Sleep Patterns: Biological, Social, and Psychological Influences*, Cambridge University Press (2002).

5 LeBourgeois, M. K., Carskadon, M. A., Akacem, L. D., Simpkin,
   C. T., Wright, K. P., Achermann, P., Jenni, O. G., 'Circadian phase
   and its relationship to nighttime sleep in toddlers', *J Biol Rhythms*,
   28(5) (2013), pp. 322–31.

6 Hunziker, U. A., Barr, R. G. , 'Increased carrying reduces infant
   crying: a randomized controlled trial', *Pediatrics*, 77(5) (1986), pp.
   641–8.

7 Morelli, G. A., Rogoff, B., Oppenheim, D., Goldsmith, D.,
   'Cultural variation in infants' sleeping arrangements: questions of
   independence', *Developmental Psychology*, 28 (1992), pp. 604–13.

8 Brazelton, T., 'Parent-infant co-sleeping revisited', *Ab Initio.*, 2(1)
   (1990).

9 Fukumizu, M., Kaga, M., Kohyama, J., Hayes, M. J., 'Sleep-related
   nighttime crying (yonaki) in Japan: a community-based study',
   Pediatrics, 115(1) (2005), pp. 217–24.

10 Kohyama, J., Mindell, J. A., Sadeh, A., 'Sleep characteristics of
   young children in Japan: internet study and comparison with
   other Asian countries', *Pediatr Int.*, 53(5) (2011), pp. 649–55.

11 Mindell, J. A. , Sadeh, A., Kwon, R., Goh, D. Y., 'Cross-cultural
   comparison of maternal sleep', *Sleep*, 36(11) (2013), pp. 1699–706.

12 Mindell, J. A., Sadeh, A., Kohyama, J., How, T. H., 'Parental
   behaviors and sleep outcomes in infants and toddlers: a cross-
   cultural comparison', *Sleep Med.*, 11(4) (2010), pp. 393–9.

13 Worthman, C. M., Brown, R. A., 'Sleep budgets in a globalizing
   world: biocultural interactions influence sleep sufficiency among
   Egyptian families', *Soc Sci Med.*, 79 (2013), pp. 31–9.

14 Worthman, C. M., Brown, R. A., 'Companionable sleep: social
   regulation of sleep and cosleeping in Egyptian families', *J Fam
   Psychol.*, 21(1) (2007), pp. 124–35.

Chapter 4

1 Jenness, R., 'The composition of human milk', *Semin Perinatol.*,
   3(3) (1979), pp. 225–39.

2 Vennemann, M. M., Bajanowski, T., Brinkmann, B., Jorch, G.,
   Yücesan, K., Sauerland, C., Mitchell, E. A., 'Does breastfeeding
   reduce the risk of sudden infant death syndrome?', *Pediatrics*,
   123(3) (2009), pp. 406–10.

3   Montgomery-Downs, H. E., Clawges, H. M., Santy, E. E., 'Infant feeding methods and maternal sleep and daytime functioning', *Pediatrics*, 126(6) (2010), pp. 1562–8.

4   Cohen Engler, A., Hadash, A., Shehadeh, N., Pillar, G., 'Breastfeeding may improve nocturnal sleep and reduce infantile colic: potential role of breast milk melatonin', *Eur J Pediatr.*, 171(4) (2012), pp. 729–32.

5   Keane, V. et al., 'Do solids help baby sleep through the night?', *Am J Dis Child, 142*(1988), pp. 404–5; Macknin, M. L., Medendorp, S. V., Maier, M. C., 'Infant sleep and bedtime cereal', *Am J Dis Child*, 143(9) (1989), pp. 1066–8.

6   Foote, K. D., Marriott, L. D., 'Weaning of infants', *Arch Dis Child*, 88 (2003), pp. 488–92.

7   Hartmann, E., 'Effects of L-tryptophan on sleepiness and on sleep', *Journal Psychiatric Research*, 17(2) (1982), pp. 107–13.

8   Rowe, K. S., Rowe, K. J., 'Synthetic food coloring and behavior: a dose response effect in a double-blind, placebo-controlled, repeated-measures study', *J Pediatr.*, 125(5 Pt 1) (1994), pp. 691–8.

9   Kaplan, B. J., McNicol, J., Conte, R. A., Moghadam, H. K., 'Dietary replacement in preschool-aged hyperactive boys', *Pediatrics*, 83(1) (1989), pp. 7–17.

10 Fitzsimon, M., Holborow, P., Berry, P., Latham, S., 'Salicylate sensitivity in children reported to respond to salicylate exclusion', *Med J Aust.*, 2(12) (1978), pp. 570–2.

11 Kahn, A., Mozin, M. J., Casimir, G., Montauk, L., Blum, D., 'Insomnia and cow's milk allergy in infants', *Pediatrics*, 76(6) (1985), pp. 880–4.

12 Jamison, J. R., Davies, N. J., 'Chiropractic management of cow's milk protein intolerance in infants with sleep dysfunction syndrome: a therapeutic trial', *J Manipulative Physiol Ther.*, 29(6) (2006), pp. 469–74.

13 Montgomery, P. et al., 'Fatty acids and sleep in UK children: Subjective and pilot objective sleep results from the DOLAB study – a randomised controlled trial', *Journal of Sleep Research*, March 2014.

Chapter 5

1   Middlemiss, W., Granger, D. A. , Goldberg, W. A., Nathans, L., 'Asynchrony of mother-infant hypothalamic-pituitary-adrenalaxis activity following extinction of infant crying responses induced during the transition to sleep', *Early Hum Dev.*, 88(4) (2012), pp. 227–32.

2   Douglas, P. S., Hill, P. S., 'Behavioral sleep interventions in the first six months of life do not improve outcomes for mothers or infants: a systematic review', *J Dev Behav Pediatr.*, 34(7) (2013), pp. 497–507.

3   Price, A., Wake, M., Ukoumunne, O., Hiscock, H., 'Five-year follow-up of harms and benefits of behavioral infant sleep intervention: randomized trial', *Pediatrics,* (2012) Published online 10 Sept 2012.

Chapter 6

1   Jenni, O. G., Fuhrer, H. Z., Iglowstein, I., Molinari, L., Largo, R. H., 'A longitudinal study of bed sharing and sleep problems among Swiss children in the first 10 years of life', *Pediatrics*, 115(1) (2005), pp. 233–40.

2   Okami, P., Weisner, T., Olmstead, R., 'Outcome correlates of parent-child bedsharing: an eighteen-year longitudinal study', *J Dev Behav Pediatr.,* 23(4) (2002), pp. 244–53.

3   Barajas, R. G., Martin, A., Brooks-Gunn, J., Hale, L., 'Mother-child bedsharing in toddlerhood and cognitive and behavioral outcomes', *Pediatrics,* 128(2) (2011), pp. 339–47.

4   Olsen, N. J., Pedersen, J., Händel, M. N., Stougaard, M., Mortensen, E. L., Heitmann, B. L., 'Child behavioural problems and body size among 2-6 year old children predisposed to overweight. Results from the "healthy start" study', *PloS One*, 8(11) (2013).

5   Blair, P., Heron, J., Fleming, P., 'Relationship between bed sharing and breastfeeding: longitudinal, population-based analysis', *Pediatrics* (2010) 10.1542/peds.2010–277.

6   Ibid.

7   Horne, R. S., Parslow, P. M., Ferens, D., Watts, A. M., Adamson, T. M., 'Comparison of evoked arousability in breast and formula fed infants', *Arch Dis Child*, 89(1) (2004), pp. 22–5.

8 Mindell, J. A., Telofski, L. S., Wiegand, B., Kurtz, E. S., 'A nightly bedtime routine: impact on sleep in young children and maternal mood', *J Fam Psychol.*, 25(3) (2011), pp. 423–33.

9 Ibid.

10 Shinkoda, H. et al., 'Analysis of parent-child sleeping and living habits related to later bedtimes in children', *Fukuoka Igaku Zasshi*, 103(1) (2012), pp. 12–23.

11 Deakin, A., 'Children's choice of comforters and their effects on sleep', *Br J Community Nurs.*, 9(3) (2004), pp. 126–30.

12 Caldwell, B. A., Redeker, N. S., 'Maternal stress and psychological status and sleep in minority preschool children', *Public Health Nurs.*, 6 Jan 2014.

13 Teti, D. M., Crosby, B. 'Maternal depressive symptoms, dysfunctional cognitions, and infant night waking: the role of maternal nighttime behaviour', *Child Dev.*, 83(3) (2012), pp. 939–53.

14 Dennis, C. L., Ross, L., 'Relationships among infant sleep patterns, maternal fatigue, and development of depressive symptomatology', *Birth*, 32(3) (2005), pp. 187–93.

15 Waters, S. F., West, T. V., Mendes, W. B., 'Stress contagion physiological covariation between mothers and infants', *Psychological Science*, 30 Jan 2014.

16 Harrison, Y., 'The relationship between daytime exposure to light and night-time sleep in 6-12 week old infants', *J Sleep Res.*, 13(4) (2004), pp. 345–52.

17 Field, T., Cullen, C., Largie, S., Diego, M., Schanberg, S., Kuhn, C., 'Lavender bath oil reduces stress and crying and enhances sleep in very young infants', *Early Hum Dev.*, 84(6) (2008), pp. 399–401.

18 Çetinkaya, B., Başbakkal, Z., 'The effectiveness of aromatherapy massage using lavender oil as a treatment for infantile colic', *Int J Nurs Pract.*, 18(2) (2012), pp. 164–9.

19 Goel, N., Kim, H., Lao, R. P., 'An olfactory stimulus modifies nighttime sleep in young men and women', *Chronobiol Int.*, 22(5) (2005), pp. 889–904.

20 Loewy, J., Hallan, C., Friedman, E., Martinez, C., 'Sleep/sedation in children undergoing EEG testing: a comparison of chloral hydrate and music therapy', *Am J Electroneurodiagnostic Technol.*, 46(4) (2006), pp. 343–55.

21 Tan, L. P., 'The effects of background music on quality of sleep in elementary school children', *J Music Ther.*, 41(2) (2004), pp. 128–50.

Chapter 7

1   Hunziker, U. A., Barr, R. G., 'Increased carrying reduces infant crying: a randomized controlled trial', *Pediatrics,* 77(5) (1986), pp. 641–8.

2   Gerard, C. M., Harris, K. A., Thach, B. T., 'Spontaneous arousals in supine infants while swaddled and unswaddled during rapid eye movement and quiet sleep', *Pediatrics*, 110(6) (2002), p. 70.

3   Gessner, B. D., Ives, G. C., Perham-Hester, K. A., 'Association between sudden infant death syndrome and prone sleep position, bed sharing, and sleeping outside an infant crib in Alaska', *Pediatrics*, 108(4) (2001), pp. 923–7.

4   Jeffery, H. E., Megevand, A., Page, H. D., 'Why the prone position is a risk factor for sudden infant death syndrome', *Pediatrics*, 104(2 Pt 1) (1999), pp. 263–9.

5   St James-Roberts, I., Alvarez, M., Csipke, E., Abramsky, T., Goodwin, J., Sorgenfrei, E., 'Infant crying and sleeping in London, openhagen and when parents adopt a "proximal" form of care', *Pediatrics*, 117(6) (2006), e1146–55.

6   Varendi, H., Christensson, K., Porter, R. H., Winberg, J., 'Soothing effect of amniotic fluid smell in newborn infants', *Early Hum Dev.*, 51(1) (1998), pp. 47–55.

7   Porter, R. H., Winberg, J., 'Unique salience of maternal breast odors for newborn infants', *Neurosci Biobehav Rev.*, 23(3) (1999), pp. 439–49.

8   Galland, B. C., Taylor, B. J., Elder, D. E., Herbison, P., 'Normal sleep patterns in infants and children: a systematic review of observational studies', *Sleep Med Rev.*, 16(3) (2012), pp. 213–22.

9   Ibid.

10 Michelsson, K., Rinne, A., Paajanen, S. 'Crying, feeding and sleeping patterns in 1 to 12-month-old infants', *Child Care Health Dev.*, 16(2) (1990), pp. 99–111.

11 Galland, B. C., Taylor, B. J., Elder, D. E., Herbison, P., 'Normal sleep patterns in infants and children: a systematic review of observational studies', *Sleep Med Rev.*, 16(3) (2012), pp. 213–22.

12 Michelsson, K., Rinne, A., Paajanen, S., 'Crying, feeding and sleeping patterns in 1 to 12-month-old infants', *Child Care Health Dev.*, 16(2) (1990), pp. 99–111.

13 Iglowstein, I., Jenni, O. G., Molinari, L., Largo, R. H., 'Sleep duration from infancy to adolescence: reference values and generational trends', *Pediatrics*, 111(2) (2003), pp. 302–7.

14 Henderson, J. et al., 'Sleeping through the night: the consolidation of self-regulated sleep across the first year of life', *Pediatrics*, 126(5) (2010), pp. 1081–7.

15 Scher, A., 'A longitudinal study of night waking in the first year', *Child Care Health Dev.*, 17(5) (1991), pp. 295–302.

16 Armstrong, K. L., Quinn, R. A., Dadds, M. R., 'The sleep patterns of normal children', *Med J Aust.*, 161(3) (1994), pp. 202–6.

17 Iglowstein, I., Jenni, O. G., Molinari, L., Largo, R. H., 'Sleep duration from infancy to adolescence: Reference values and generational trends, *Pediatrics*, 111(2) (2003), pp. 302–7.

Chapter 8

1 Burnham, M. M., Goodlin-Jones, B. L., Gaylor, E. E. and Anders, T. F., 'Nighttime sleep-wake patterns and self-soothing from birth to one year of age: a longitudinal intervention study', *J Child Psychol Psychiatry*, 43(6) (2002), pp. 713–25.

2 Price, A. M., Brown, J. E., Bittman, M., Wake, M., Quach, J., Hiscock, H., 'Children's sleep patterns from 0 to 9 years: Australian population longitudinal study', *Arch Dis Child*, 99(2) (2014), pp. 119–25.

3 Armstrong, K. L., Quinn, R. A. and Dadds, M. R., 'The sleep patterns of normal children', *Medical Journal of Australia*, 161(3) (1994), pp. 202–6.

4 Sadler, S., 'Sleep: what is normal at six months?', *Prof Care Mother Child*, 4(6) (1994), pp. 166–7.

5 Wake, M., Hesketh, K., Lucas, J., 'Teething and tooth eruption in infants: A cohort study', *Pediatrics*, 106(6) (2000), pp. 1374–9; Owais, A. I., Zawaideh, F., Bataineh, O., 'Challenging parents' myths regarding their children's teething', *Int J Dent Hyg.*, 8(4) (2010), p. 324.

Chapter 9

1   Sadler, S., 'Sleep: what is normal at six months?', *Prof Care Mother Child*, 4(6) (1994), pp. 166–7.

2   Armstrong, K. L., Quinn, R. A. and Dadds, M. R., 'The sleep patterns of normal children', *Medical Journal of Australia*, 161(3) (1994), pp. 202–6.

3   Ibid.

Chapter 10

1   Armstrong, K. L., Quinn, R. A. and Dadds, M. R., 'The sleep patterns of normal children', *Medical Journal of Australia*, 161(3) (1994), pp. 202–6.

2   Scher, A., 'A longitudinal study of night waking in the first year', *Child Care Health Dev.*, 17(5) (1991), pp. 295–302.

3   Goodlin-Jones, B. L. et al., 'Night waking, sleep-wake organization, and self-soothing in the first year of life', *J Dev Behav Pediatr.*, 22(4) (2001), pp. 226–33.

4   Armstrong, K. L., Quinn, R. A., Dadds, M. R., 'The sleep patterns of normal children', *Medical Journal of Australia,* 161(3) (1994), pp. 202–6.

Chapter 12

1   Scher, A., 'A longitudinal study of night waking in the first year', *Child Care Health Dev.*, 17(5) (1991), pp. 295–302.

Index